Clinical Judgement in the Health and Welfare Professions

Extending the evidence base

Clinical Judgement in the Health and Welfare Professions

Extending the evidence base

Susan White and John Stancombe

Open University Press
Maidenhead · Philadelphia

Open University Press
McGraw-Hill Education
McGraw-Hill House
Shoppenhangers Road
Maidenhead
Berkshire
England
SL6 2QL

email: enquiries@openup.co.uk
world wide web: www.openup.co.uk

and
325 Chestnut Street
Philadelphia, PA 19106, USA

First Published 2003

A catalogue record of this book is available from the British Library

ISBN 0 335 20874 6 (pb) 0 335 20875 4 (hb)

Library of Congress Cataloging-in-Publication Data

White, Susan, 1961–
    Clinical judgement in the health and welfare professions: extending the evidence base/Susan White and John Stancombe.
        p. cm.
    Includes bibliographical references and index.
    ISBN 0–335–20875–4 (hbk.) – ISBN 0–335–20874–6 (pbk.)
    1. Medical logic. 2. Evidence-based medicine. I. Stancombe, John, 1957–II. Title.
    R723. W465 2003
    616–dc21

                                                                    2002035545

Typeset by RefineCatch Limited, Bungay, Suffolk
Printed in Great Britain by Biddles Ltd, *www.biddles.co.uk*

Contents

Preface   viii

Acknowledgements   xii

PART 1
Theorizing Clinical Judgement   1

1   Science and art   3
Approaches to understanding clinical judgement
     Practically Popper? The clinician as everyday scientist   5
     The practical problems with Popper   6
     Tackling error: the clinician and cognitive (in)competence   8
     The relationship between the knower and the known   14
     The artfulness of science and the science of artfulness   16
     Summary   22

2   Seductive certainties   24
The 'scientific-bureaucratic' model
     Political pragmatism: the ascent of scientific-bureaucratic
     rationality   26
     What is wrong with evidence-based practice?   28
     The Enlightenment: reason, progress and science   33
     Shaking the certainty   34
     Clinical judgement and different kinds   37
     Summary   39

3   Interrogating the tacit dimension   40
Concepts and methods
     The humanities and humaneness   41
     Psychoanalysis and self-knowledge   42
     Interpretive social science and the sociology of everyday life   44
     Deep familiarity: the ethnographic case study   49
     Ordinary action: ethnomethodology and conversation analysis   51
     Membership categorization: talking morality   55
     Storytelling in clinical practice: discourse studies   58
     Summary   60

PART 2
Being Realistic about Clinical Judgement: Case Formulation in Context   61

4   Clinical science as social practice   63
    Using formal knowledge in professional work
        From laboratory to clinic: producing and distributing science   64
        Looking and learning? Observation in practice   68
        Reading and interpreting the body: journal science in action?   69
        Beyond 'knowledge to go?' Popular knowledge and clinical
        practice   78
        Reading relationships: psychological theory and observation   80
        Summary   90

5   Emotion and morality   91
    Blameworthiness, creditworthiness and clinical judgement
        Good patients/bad patients   93
        Moral judgements and organizational context   95
        Moral judgements and child health: invoking parental love   98
        Privileging the child's voice: negotiating blame in interaction   102
        Producing moral selves: getting the job done   108
        Contesting moral selves: blame and moral judgement in
        multidisciplinary work   110
        Summary   112

6   Science, morality and case formulation in paediatrics   114
    A case study
        The problematics of case formulation in paediatrics   114
        The natural and the social: 'not just medical' cases   116
        Summary   128

7   Managing multiple versions   130
    Rhetoric and moral judgement in a family therapy case
        The moral context of family work   131
        Doing neutrality in talk with families: the first paradox   133
        Making knowledge and performing clinical judgement: the second
        paradox   136
        Moving from backstage to frontstage: the third paradox   138
        Summary   143

8   Clinical judgement in context   145
    Towards a more realistic realism
        Misunderstanding science: why we don't need the 'science wars'   148
        Can EBP provide protection from fashion and fad?   151

Sociological inquiry: some uses and abuses   153
Connecting research with the swampy lowlands of practice   155
Developing reflexivity: beyond reflection on action   156
Beyond training: educating judgement   159

Appendix: Transcription conventions   163

Glossary   164

Recommended further reading   169

References   174

Index   187

Preface

This book examines how professionals practising in various health and welfare settings go about the ordinary, but complicated, business of making sense of the symptoms and troubles with which their patients or clients present. Our motivations for writing the book are varied, but are the result of our conversations with each other about the problem of judgement in clinical practice, which have taken place over many years of professional, academic and research collaboration. We share a practice background in child health and welfare services, but also an academic interest in the importance of language and social interaction in human life. There is a complex dialogue, and at times an inevitable tension, between the conceptual frameworks derived from the study of everyday talk and work and the pragmatic day-to-day business of getting clinical work done. Our experience of these dialogues and tensions has inspired us to convince others that the understandings that result may help them to think about their work in new and interesting ways.

This recasting of practice is particularly important in the current policy climate. In the past decade, the problem of clinical judgement has become reduced to the simple question 'What works?' Codified knowledge in various forms has come to be defined as a safe and secure base for professional judgements. Such knowledge is ostensibly insulated from and uncontaminated by the contingencies and errors of everyday practice. While we certainly do not wish to suggest that the efficacy and safety of treatments and interventions is in any way unimportant, it does lead to a conspicuous neglect of other areas of clinical activity. Before they can begin to think about 'What works?' clinicians must first address the question 'What's wrong?', or 'What sort of problem is this?' Yet the complex processes by which professionals negotiate problem formulation remain seriously under-explored in current policy initiatives. Drawing on detailed empirical studies of everyday practice and developments in the social studies of science, we aim to convince you that clinical judgement and case formulation have important social and moral dimensions. We are not suggesting that science and evidence are not important. Such an argument would be ridiculous and quite untenable. Instead, we want to explore *how* science and evidence are used in practice. For example, how do clinicians interpret X-rays and test results? How do understandings of disease change over time and what kinds of things influence those processes? Is the science involved in clinical work different in any way from that taking place in laboratories? Is theoretical knowledge different from scientific knowledge? If so, what does this mean for practice?

Moreover, while recognizing the importance of science, we want to examine the role of other forms of reasoning, particularly that of emotion and moral judgement. For example, our work in child health and welfare services has alerted us to the importance of blame and responsibility. Our clinical experience is that accountability is a ubiquitous but frequently under-explored and tacit theme in everyday work with children and families. For example, the question of blame is often explicit right from the beginning of work with families. Parents may blame themselves or their partner for their child's 'problem'; or a young person may blame their parent for the family's troubles. Alternatively, parents may present overt accounts or explanations of their child's problem that attribute blame or responsibility to factors beyond their control. For example, a parent might attribute the problem to individual factors in the child such as difficult temperament or individual pathology, or to the inappropriate behaviour of the other parent, or to some factor in school. Thus, for one family trouble there may be many competing causal explanations, each carrying varying potential for moral censure of individual family members. However, it is not only in family work that moral judgement is important. We argue that it is a mundane feature of work in a variety of settings, including biomedicine. As such, it needs to be properly explored and debated.

In essence, this book contends that problems of judgement are intrinsic and inescapable imperatives for clinicians. Professionals are routinely faced with having to decide which diagnosis, or whose version or account of the troubles, they find most convincing and/or morally robust. In exploring these themes we have drawn on our own and others' empirical work in health and welfare settings. Many studies of professional practice are oriented to uncovering errors or abusive practices. That is, they are concerned with how work *should* be done. Our intention is different. We set out to describe how it *is* done in a variety of settings. Therefore, the studies we have drawn upon all take a descriptive approach. They seek to describe in detail the ordinary work taking place in clinics and services, rather as an anthropologist may describe the everyday practices and understandings of faraway cultures. Many of the studies make use of recordings of conversations to illustrate the way work gets done in interaction and how understandings emerge over time.

While there is an abundant literature on professional–client interaction in various settings, we have concentrated primarily on studies of interprofessional communication. We have done so because our concern is with how professionals formulate cases. Case formulations often remain unarticulated in encounters with patients and clients and may not exist as single events produced spontaneously on discrete occasions. They may, for example, emerge gradually over time or through conversations with colleagues. They may thus be at their most explicit in the conversations taking place *between* professionals (Atkinson 1995). As Anspach notes:

> Although much has been written concerning how doctors talk *to* patients, very little has been written about how doctors talk *about* patients ... This analytic focus on the medical interview occurs even though the way in which physicians talk about patients is a potentially valuable source of information about medical culture. Rarely do doctors reveal their assumptions about patients when they are talking to them.
>
> (Anspach 1988: 358)

We should say a little more at this point about our own studies, from which many of the extracts are taken. The examples from paediatric and child psychiatry services are taken from White's study of an integrated child health service situated in a district general hospital in the North of England (White 2002). The service comprises paediatric inpatient and outpatient, child and adolescent mental health (CAMHS), child development (CDS) and social work services. Together, the services provide general secondary care to a socio-economically diverse community, with tertiary specialist services provided at regional centres. Methods included observation of clinics, ward rounds and staff/team meetings, audio-recording of interprofessional talk in meetings and other less formal settings, such as before and after clinics, the tracking of a number of individual cases through the services and a documentary analysis of medical notes. Stancombe's data are taken from his study of family therapy (Stancombe 2003), which took place in a family therapy clinic within a generic child and adolescent mental health service, in a NHS trust in the north of England. The research was based on two family therapy clinics within the service. Each clinic involved a small team of therapists with a special interest in a family systems approach. They provided assessment and therapeutic services to children and families experiencing emotional and behavioural difficulties, with the majority of referrals coming from primary care sources.

In Part 1 of the book, we develop the conceptual framework. In Chapter 1, we consider the range of approaches that have been used to explain and explore clinical judgement, or more particularly case formulation. In Chapter 2, we examine current policy initiatives and some of their intended and unintended consequences. We explore some of the historical and philosophical antecedents for the current preoccupation with rational–technical forms of reasoning. Chapter 3 reviews a range of frameworks that can be used to open up the areas of practice that are neglected in more traditional approaches. We build a case for the use of the various methodologies associated with interpretive social science as a means to examine what is taken for granted in professional activity. In particular, we introduce the different ways in which various academic and philosophical traditions have analysed talk and text and give some examples of empirical work relevant to clinical judgement.

In Part 2 of the book, we apply the ideas from earlier chapters to particular kinds of professional reasoning. Chapter 4 examines how scientific and theoretical ideas are used in practice. It seeks to challenge two misconceptions: first, that science inevitably reduces uncertainty; second, that less conventionally scientific domains of practice, such as therapeutics and social care, are necessarily riddled with uncertainty. We argue that professionals often accomplish certainty by using moral judgements and personal experience and by engaging in artful rhetoric and persuasion. In Chapter 5, we consider the moral dimensions of clinical judgement, arguing not only that moral reasoning is inexorably bound to case formulation in many settings, but also that professionals must construct themselves as moral actors in various kinds of ways. Chapters 6 and 7 provide more detailed case examples taken from our own research. Chapter 6 explores the many different kinds of reasoning used in the formulation of a difficult paediatric case. Chapter 7, using a family therapy case, examines critically the idea that moral neutrality is possible. In the final chapter we build a case for a more 'realistic' approach to understanding clinical judgement, which paradoxically acknowedges that case formulation is a messy business that is often subjective and relative, and resolutely depends on language, persuasion and emotion. We draw out some implications of these observations for research, practice and professional education.

Finally, we should note that the studies we have cited often draw on ideas that may be unfamiliar to many readers. We have endeavoured to make these accessible to practitioners. However, there is a danger in any such translation that ideas become decontextualized and oversimplified. Obviously, this oversimplification obscures as much as it reveals and can thus create considerable confusion if people want to build on their understandings in future reading. Therefore, we have tried to strike a balance between achieving accessibility and preserving the integrity of the relevant conceptual frameworks. However, to assist the reader, we have provided a glossary of key terms and a brief annotated guide to further reading at the end of the book.

Acknowledgements

We should like to acknowledge the contribution to the production of this book of a number of people, including the clinicians whose words we have represented in the chapters that follow. We hope they will feel that we have adequately illustrated the complex nature of their work. Sue would especially like to thank her family, Alex, Joe and Tom, for their tolerance of her intense relationship with the computer, her mother Jenny for bridging some of the domestic gaps and her friend Mary Dover for being Mary. John would particularly like to thank Ruth, Joe, Kieran and Ella for their help and understanding during the writing up of his research and Stephen Frosh for his constructive comments throughout.

We are both most grateful to Angus Clarke, who has provided invaluable advice on a number of clinical issues. Thanks also go to Carolyn Taylor for her support, her comments on the chapters and for being one of the most widely read people alive and hence an indispensable source of references on a host of topics. Sue White's research was supported by the Economic and Social Research Council (research grant number R000222892).

PART 1
Theorizing Clinical Judgement

1 Science and art
Approaches to understanding clinical judgement

> Clinicians are determinists in their diagnostic activities. That is, symptoms, signs and the like are viewed as manifestations of underlying causal processes that can be known in principle. Because much clinical reasoning involves diagnosis or backward inference (i.e. making inferences from effects to prior causes), the clinician, like the historian, has much latitude (or degrees of freedom) in reconstructing the past to make the present seem most likely.
>
> (Einhorn 1988: 182)

This book is about case formulation. It is about how health and welfare professionals make sense of the problems and needs of the people who come to their services, how they build formulations about what has caused these 'troubles' and how they decide what should be done about them. It examines how clinicians and practitioners exercise their 'degrees of freedom' in making sense of cases and what the limits of these freedoms are. Clearly, the judgements made in the course of clinical activity really matter. Once crafted as case formulations, they travel through time and space and carry serious consequences. In short, people are directly affected by the constructions and reconstructions of 'the problem' that constitute professional judgement. It is no surprise, therefore, that there is already an abundant and eclectic literature on professional reasoning, much of which originates in the relatively esoteric domains of mathematics and cognitive psychology. This literature focuses particularly on the flaws, biases and errors in clinicians' judgements and how they should be remedied.

Our own approach to case formulation and clinical judgement is a little different and draws principally on **ethnographic** and **discourse analytic** studies of professional work. We have taken this focus precisely because such studies look at the detail of what clinicians actually do, what they say and what they write in the course of their day-to-day activity. This detail facilitates the examination of clinical judgement in context and allows a proper acknowledgement of its complexity. In Chapter 3, we say more about why we think this particular approach and the understandings it can yield are important for practitioners. However, first we need to summarize the existing literature on clinical judgement and raise some questions about the sorts of assumptions and priorities that have driven particular models.

The literature on clinical judgement is dominated by analyses of medical decision-making. This provokes particular interest because the rapid technological and biomedical advances of the second half of the twentieth century have expanded the repertoire of available judgements at an unprecedented rate, and have increased the possibility that choices made by clinicians may retrospectively be constructed as errors. However, while biomedicine is the focus of much of the literature, it is important to note that many of the assumptions have been exported to other health and welfare contexts.

Our review of the existing literature is necessarily brief. The field is vast and can be grouped and ordered in any number of ways. An exhaustive exploration would run to several volumes and the summary we provide here carries its own arbitrariness. We have given some suggestions for further reading at the end of the book. The ideas we present should not in any way be seen on a progressive continuum. One form of understanding has not superseded or silenced the others (Berg 1997); instead they all continue to circulate as competing accounts of how judgements are made and/or how they *should* be made.

Clinical practice has a complex relationship to science and scientific method. For example, doctors and professions allied to medicine rely on the sciences of anatomy, physiology, pharmacology, pathology, genetics and so forth in their work, but the business of clinical judgement has also traditionally been seen as 'scientific' in character. For example, many health and welfare professionals rely on formal classifications and categorizations, which help them to order and make sense of their cases. The most obvious examples of these are the systems for the classification of disease (**nosologies**) used in biomedicine. However, like scientists, clinicians in all settings are also involved in the generation of causal *explanations* for the symptoms, or troubles they encounter in their work.

So what sort of scientific method has become most associated with the process of generating explanations and judgements in clinical encounters? Clinical judgement is a peculiar science. Even when it is based on the application of the *relatively* stable sciences of biomedicine, rarely can it rely on clear sets of causal laws leading in any straightforward way to a specific conclusion or solution. Clinical judgement is not and never can be Euclidean geometry. Instead, it is generally characterized by shifting formulations, carrying varying 'degrees of confidence' (Little 1995). At any given time, then, there may be any number of potentially competent interpretations (or competing hypotheses) about a particular case. Thus, it has been argued, the form of reasoning in competent clinical judgement should bear a close relationship to a version of scientific method known as the **hypothetico-deductive method**, derived from the work of Karl Popper (1959), an influential scientist and philosopher of science.

Practically Popper? The clinician as everyday scientist

The hypothetico-deductive method works through a process of falsification. The idea is that, by conducting a rigorous search for disconfirming evidence, the clinician works successively to disprove each of the competing hypotheses about the symptom or trouble, so that the hypothesis with the 'best fit' will ultimately prove most robust. The routine practice in medicine of generating 'differential diagnoses' (or competing causal explanations) for presenting problems may be seen as an example of the adaptation of principles of the hypothetico-deductive method for day-to-day pragmatic use. The method is also frequently advocated as a 'gold standard' of good practice in the more 'fuzzy' and contested areas of clinical judgement, such as psychotherapy and social care (for example, Snyder and Thomsen 1988; Turk *et al.* 1988; Sheppard 1995, 1998), which have less stable knowledge bases. For example, Sheppard makes the following observations about social work assessments:

> Poor practice is marked by a lack of clarity in hypothesis formulation. The search for disconfirming evidence is made difficult by the difficulty in identifying what it is that is being disconfirmed . . . Sensitivity to disconfirming evidence has two dimensions. First, it is possible for a practitioner to proceed in a manner which seeks to confirm initial impressions or preconceived ideas . . . The second relates to evidence, although collected during assessment, which, because it contradicts explicit or implicit hypotheses, is ignored.
>
> (Sheppard 1995: 278–9)

The basic tenets of the hypothetico-deductive method can be summarized as follows:

1 The better version is out there to be found and by following a series of logical reasoning processes we shall be able to find it.
2 These reasoning processes should aim to be rational-cognitive and 'objectivized'.
3 Competing explanations and frameworks are generally mutually exclusive – only one can be 'more true', at any one time.

Clearly, the hypothetico-deductive method implies a rational, objective, linear process and in certain circumstances it has much to commend it, but it has also has some serious limitations as a typology of professional decision-making.

The practical problems with Popper

The straightforward application of the hypothetico-deductive method to the process of clinical judgement is problematic in a number of ways. For example, the encounters between professional or clinician and their patient/client and the subsequent conversations between the clinician and his or her colleagues are conducted through language and there is ample room for misunderstanding, incomplete versions and false trails, as Little notes:

> Whether doctors know it or not, there is always the possibility of confusion in consultations because of the linguistic habits of both doctors and patients, unintentionally used in the way they speak to each other. Each party attaches certain meanings to words and phrases and assumes that the meaning is understood by the other party – who may in fact hear the word or phrase and attach quite a different meaning to it.
>
> (Little 1995: 145)

Moreover, more than one hypothesis may be true at the same time. For example, patients consulting a physician or surgeon might present with symptoms that might have multiple causes – finding a 'fit' for one hypothesis does not necessarily eliminate the validity of the others.

In the social care field things are even more complicated. For example, in the context of social work, Sheppard (1995) supports his arguments with a case study, which is used to illustrate the process of progressive hypothesis development. It begins as follows:

> A 14-year-old may be referred by his ... parents because he is disobedient and close to being 'out of control' ... The parents may themselves present this as a personality issue: this is an awkward life stage and a nasty egocentric boy.

Sheppard suggests that initial interviews show the boy to be 'sensitive' and the preliminary hypothesis (the parents' version) to be incorrect, and hence we must look to other frameworks for an alternative. He continues:

the father and mother have been arguing frequently, and this relates
to poor performance of her traditional (maternal) role ... We
may then hypothesize that the woman is depressed because she
feels trapped within the limits of her traditional role expectations.
Although the boy's problems cannot be ignored, the central problem
is in fact the mother's depression, arising from her individual
experience of oppression.

(Sheppard 1995: 276)

Of course, this may well be so but, as White (1997a) argues, there is nothing
in this description of the case to 'prove' or even strongly suggest that the
'maternal depression' hypothesis has the best fit. It is equally possible to see
the mother's depression as a result of her attempts to deal with a recalcitrant
teenage child who is 'nasty and egocentric' at home but charming to strangers,
or as a series of circular hypotheses, with each causing the other in an endless
loop. This leads White (1997a) to argue that there may be 'equally valid'
versions of the same phenomenon and that sometimes there are no neutral
mechanisms for making a choice between those versions. So the hypothetico-
deductive method has limitations in dealing with ambiguity, complexity and
often intractable uncertainty.

However, there is also some evidence that the hypothetico-deductive
method may not be the best way of understanding the processes of clinical
judgement in cases which are relatively straightforward and certain. For
example, during routine clinical encounters involving familiar non-complex
cases, experienced practitioners appear to make little or no explicit use of
hypotheses (*inter alia*, Groen and Patel 1985; Brooks *et al.* 1991; Eva *et al.*
1998; Elstein and Schwartz 2000). Under such conditions, they rely on their
knowledge of the particular domain, and of other similar cases they have
encountered: 'Once a physician has seen a case of chicken pox, it is a relatively
simple matter to diagnose the next case by recalling the characteristic appearance of the rash' (Elstein and Schwartz 2000: 97). Rather than generating
unnecessary sets of competing hypotheses, it is suggested that clinicians
in such circumstances rely on 'pattern recognition' (Groen and Patel 1985)
based on stored knowledge: 'I know this is chicken pox, because it looks like
chicken pox.'

These kinds of pattern recognition processes are evident across a range of
health and welfare professions. For example, during recent fieldwork, one of us
(White) observed a child psychiatry clinic, during which the psychiatrist
assessed a child aged eight who had been referred because of his 'odd'
behaviour. After spending 15 minutes observing this child and speaking to
him, the psychiatrist said very firmly, 'This is Asperger's [Syndrome]' (a
social communication disorder often described as a mild form of autism).
However, on many other occasions, this same psychiatrist arrived at such

diagnoses only following lengthy assessments and sometimes considerable debate with different professionals involved. Because this particular child presented with 'classical' features, the psychiatrist immediately, spontaneously and apparently with complete certainty assigned him to the diagnostic category 'Asperger's'. This rapid movement from data to diagnosis is labelled by Groen and Patel (1985) as forward reasoning. The literature suggests that clinicians seem to use the 'backwards reasoning' of the hypothetico-deductive method in more difficult cases, as defined and experienced by them (Norman *et al.* 1994; Davidoff 1998). So it is proposed that novices rely rather more on hypothesis generation and testing than do experienced practitioners (Elstein 1994).

Thus, while the hypothetico-deductive strategy remains central to analyses of clinical judgement, it has increasingly been criticized on the grounds that it gives an incomplete understanding of the processes involved, and because it underestimates both certainty and uncertainty in day-to-day decision-making. It has been challenged and supplemented by other ways of thinking about and attempting to improve judgement-making. These range from various forms of statistical modelling to approaches that stress the importance of intuition, tacit knowledge, language use and practical wisdom in clinical judgement. We discuss all these approaches in due course, but begin by looking at attempts to reduce the uncertainty and the potential for human failure inherent in judgement-making. Again, the field is dominated by analyses of clinical reasoning in biomedicine and professions allied to medicine.

Tackling error: the clinician and cognitive (in)competence

The 1960s and 1970s saw the development of a number of rationalizations and standardizations, aimed at making clinicians more accountable and at remedying, or reducing, uncertainty and the possibility of error (Berg 1997). These were presented as a solution to some of the worries about practice:

> Over the past few hundred years languages have been developed for collecting and interpreting evidence (statistics), dealing with uncertainty (probability theory), synthesizing evidence and estimating outcomes (mathematics) and making decisions (economics and decision theory). These languages are not currently learned by most clinical policy makers; they should be.
>
> (Eddy 1988: 58)

Often making use of statistics, probability theory and quantitative outcome measures, these developments may be seen as the ancestors of the evidence-based practice (EBP) movement (see Chapter 2).

However, alongside these mathematical solutions, developments in psychology were also crucial in the drive to improve clinical reasoning.

> In the 1970s and 1980s, new discourses became prominent in which the scientific character of medical practice became a thoroughly *individualized* notion. Rooted in the booming field of cognitive psychology, these discourses contained an image of medical practice that perfectly fitted the profession's vision of the autonomous physician.
>
> (Berg 1997: 27)

The cognitive sciences located the processes of judgement and reasoning in the individual physician's mind. Like the statistical models, the cognitive approaches focused on the limits, constraints and unintended biases of human problem solving. The physician's mind was the locus of reasoning, but it was fundamentally flawed. Human beings, it was argued, simply had their limits as information processors.

So, while advocates of the statistical model pointed to the inadequacy of clinicians' knowledge of the basic standards of probability interpretation, the cognitive psychologists produced detailed information processing models showing a number of human idiosyncrasies and fallibilities that threatened their ability to undertake the reasoning processes associated with hypothetico-deductive models. The statistical and psychological/cognitive approaches do not divide neatly. They are frequently conflated in the literature and, indeed, in the statistical models themselves, as Berg (1997: 41) notes: 'Builders of statistical tools often co-operated closely with investigators probing the workings of the physician's mind, and they phrased their descriptions of medical practice in the same way.'

Probability and clinical judgement: Bayes' theorem and decision analysis

We have already underscored the probabilistic nature of clinical judgement across a range of settings. An assortment of models has been created to assist clinicians with the calculation of probabilities and also to emulate and improve upon other aspects of human decision-making processes. The most straightforwardly mathematical of these models is based on **Bayes' theorem**, named after Thomas Bayes, an eighteenth-century mathematician. Bayes' theorem is used clinically to calculate the probability that a member of a given population who has a given symptom also has a given disease. For our more mathematically minded readers, this is represented in the formula $P(D/S) = (P(S/D) \times P(D)/P(S)$. So,

> once you have the probability of exhibiting the disease (P(D)), the probability of having the symptom (P(S)), and the probability of having the symptom if one has the disease (P(S/D), you can calculate the chance that a member of your population with symptoms S has disease D (P(D/S)).
>
> (Berg 1997: 43)

For example, during the 1970s a team of physicians and computer scientists at the University of Leeds developed a Bayesian model to be used in assessments of patients presenting with abdominal pain. The team claimed 90 per cent accuracy using the model, compared with 80 per cent for experienced doctors relying on judgement alone, which was confirmed in subsequent studies (see, *inter alia*, de Dombal *et al.* 1972; de Dombal 1989). One can see how, in clearly defined areas of clinical diagnostics, where probabilities are available to insert into the formula, Bayes' theorem could be used to assist clinical judgement. Examples of specialities where Bayes is more widely used in routine clinical contact include clinical genetics and epidemiology, as Angus Clarke (pers. comm. 2000), a clinical geneticist, notes:

> We, in clinical genetics, do use [Bayes] regularly, occasionally in the consultation (if we are given extra information to incorporate into the calculation) but usually in advance, or in preparation of a lab report – for example, what is the chance of person X carrying cystic fibrosis with a given family history, but despite a negative lab test result (the test not being able to detect all mutations)? But we are very unusual – I cannot think of many other branches of medicine where Bayes would be used explicitly (calculated), rather than just incorporated implicitly (intuitively) into what passes for 'clinical judgement'. I know that some of the clinical epidemiologists promote its use.

Bayes' theorem has enjoyed considerable durability since the 1960s and 1970s and forms the basis for a wide range of statistical models to aid decision-making. The basic theorem has been broadened in scope by the addition of **decision analysis** to many programmes, which adapts utility theory (a cost–benefit estimation derived from economics) to clinical judgement. Proponents of decision analysis argue that, by concentrating on probabilities, Bayes fails to incorporate any value judgements about the risks and benefits of particular interventions, despite the very real importance of these in real-life clinical situations. For example, Bayes may help with the diagnosis of a particular condition that would normally be treated surgically, but it will not help with the decision about whether this particular patient would benefit more from the surgery than from no intervention at all. So, whereas Bayes' theorem idealizes *objective* probabilities derived from epidemiological studies of populations or samples of patients, decision analysis makes use of *subjective* probabilities. Subjective probabilities are judgements about what, on the basis of their experience, the clinician thinks are the likely costs or benefits in a given situation. Decision analysis also includes an estimate of the patient's subjective preferences about treatment (also known as utilities).

There is little doubt that, in biomedicine and allied professions, these have proved useful and the evidence-based practice movement is fuelling their popularity. However, the tools have some shortcomings in clinical practice situations, as Angus Clarke (pers. comm. 2000) notes:

> I doubt if an average junior hospital doctor does a Bayesian calcula-tion to interpret a cardiac enzyme result on someone presenting with atypical chest pain (is this person having a heart attack?). I don't think the data would be there to permit this sum . . . What is crucial is that we simply do not know the prior probabilities in so much of clinical practice. If we look at the atypical chest pain case, for example, we might be able to generate prior probabilities (of having a MI [myocardial infarction]) for all cases of atypical chest pain that reach hospital lumped together, but that does not help with *this particular patient*, who has pain of just *this* sort rather than the more usual (more typical) atypical chest pain.

The problems of interpretation are amplified when subjective probabilities (estimates of likely benefit) are added to the sum, as Little notes:

> At a meeting on decision theory, I took part in an exercise which examined amputation of the leg for diabetic small vessel disease. The analysis by the lecturer was immaculate in its formal structure, but it reached a result diametrically opposed to my own solution, because the lecturer used a value for his assessment of quality of life after amputation which was quite unlike the one that I developed after years of work with amputees. I do not know what the 'right' answer was.
>
> (Little 1995: 71–2)

So there is a curious paradox in the statistical approaches. They seek to replace the judgements of clinicians with statistical programmes, but do not take into account the point that statistical reasoning itself requires judge-ments. The assumptions implied by statistical tools – that the values required are both neutral and knowable – are often violated by the realities of clinical practice. That is, 'information' is constructed as a neutral phenomenon (Atkinson 1995), when frequently, in practice, it is ambiguous and must be interpreted, involving the exercise of judgement (see Chapter 4). Moreover, many people coming to health and welfare services give 'poor' histories, cover up symptoms, seek to hide information that they think may expose them to blame or ridicule, have undiscovered ailments or have more than one disease at the same time. This makes statistical models difficult to apply and probably irrelevant. As Little (1995: 65) notes:

> All too often . . . clinicians work under a veil of ignorance . . . They may have to act without clear direction from their own subjective probabilities for each [possible] diagnosis because the penalties for inaction in the face of each possible diagnosis are too great. A young immuno-suppressed person dying in an intensive care unit from adult respiratory distress syndrome may be suffering from over-whelming septicaemia, endotoxaemia or cytomegalovirus infection, among many other possibilities. Such a patient will receive multiple modes of treatment because death will soon follow unless the triggering cause can be reversed.

However, not all statistical models rely solely on the fairly limited repertoire of probabilities and utilities. Social judgement theory, or **judgement analysis**, is derived from the theoretical model developed during the 1940s and 1950s by psychologist Egon Brunswick (see Cooksey 1996 for a detailed summary of this work), which located the thinking organism within an 'ecology' or environment. For Brunswick, judgements about the world would always be mediated by various situational 'cues'. These processes can be represented as statistical formulae. This model has been developed and adapted for the study of clinical judgement.

Judgement analysis takes a descriptive approach to the understanding of clinical reasoning. It examines clinicians' (judges') judgement-making 'policy' and then creates a statistical representation of that 'policy'. These statistical representations of 'policy' are also used to generate predictions allegedly more accurate than the judges' own unassisted predictions about the same case(s), because they are not affected by judgemental inconsistencies, caused by, for example, tiredness or mood. This is known as 'judgemental bootstrapping', and it has been used in a variety of service settings. For example, in a study of clinical psychologists' categorizations of patients as either neurotic or psychotic, Goldberg (1970) used equations representing the judgements of 29 psychologists to generate predictions of undiagnosed patients. He concluded: 'linear regression models of clinical judges can be more accurate diagnostic predictors than the humans who are modelled.' (Goldberg 1970: 430).

Judgement analysis begins from a descriptive rather than prescriptive/ evaluative position. It is concerned with how clinicians decide, rather than how they *should* decide. However, the models so generated have been used to highlight the alleged 'inferiority' of unaided human decision-making. Here, as in the decision analysis frameworks, inconsistency is equated with error. The statistical models, then, become the templates against which the clinician's own reasoning strategies are judged. So

> The statistical tools or expert systems were not called upon to fix some pre-given, long-since-recognized flaws in the physician's performance. Rather, these tools provided the metaphors for the working and failing of the physician's mind in the first place.
>
> (Berg 1997: 77)

Ways to stray: the deficit models

Perhaps the most influential product of the cognitive revolution in judgement analysis has been the catalogue of 'ways to stray' (Fischoff and Beyth-Marom 1988) from the ideals constructed by rational technical analyses of clinical reasoning. The built-in 'deficits' of human reasoning are widely cited in professional literature across the range of health and welfare occupations and specialties. These deficits are generally presented as more or less inevitable tendencies or predispositions, produced by the fallible human brain.

As Elstein and Schwartz (2000) note, clinicians may make judgements based on 'pattern recognition', on hypothesis generation or on a combination of the two. While each might often work very well, both have been linked to particular errors. Using 'pattern recognition', such as in the chicken pox example above, may sometimes lead to premature closure on competing explanations for the phenomenon under investigation – it may lead to the clinician jumping to conclusions. However, a model of purely **inductive** reasoning where judgements follow only after exhaustive data collection may be very inefficient and unnecessary, and produce high levels of 'cognitive strain'. Thus, clinicians tend to work with a limited number of fairly 'bounded' hypotheses that seem to be the most likely explanations.

The generation of these hypotheses is, however, affected by the cognitive capacities of the clinician in two ways: it is limited by what is *available* in memory, and by 'psychological commitment' to the first hypothesis, which makes it more difficult for the clinician subsequently to revise their formulation (Dowie and Elstein 1988: 19). This is confounded by the related tendency to seek out evidence that confirms a hypothesis, rather than searching for 'disconfirming' evidence. This is known as 'confirmation bias' (Wolf *et al.* 1985) and arguably applies even if judgement is supported by statistical models, since the clinicians must always decide whether and when to apply Bayes' theorem or any other diagnostic aid. Thus, it is argued, clinicians tend to deviate little from their initial 'anchor' hypothesis (Kahneman *et al.* 1982).

That is, they interpret new evidence only in ways that fit with their already existing formulations. A set of related errors have been catalogued for the interpretation and estimation of probabilities. First, like hypothesis formulation, the estimation of probability is affected by what is available in memory. Thus, diseases or diagnoses that are most memorable are most easily recalled. This, it is argued, leads to clinicians overestimating the probabilities of exotic and rare conditions at the expense of the more mundane and likely diagnoses.

So can either the 'statistical' or the 'cognitive' procedural models provide an adequate account of the complexities of clinical practice? It is certainly a truism that we cannot make judgements without the cognitive capacity so to do. Statistical models do not render the clinician redundant, since they are unable to activate themselves, elicit information from patients, adjudicate on its reliability or validity or decide which data are relevant. Clinical judgements are indeed impossible without the clinician's brain and, however 'social' our analytic focus, it is important to retain this dimension in any understanding of professional thinking (Cicourel 1999). It is perhaps helpful, therefore, for clinicians to have access to the rather pessimistic body of work on 'ways to stray' so that they can more rigorously monitor their own judgements.

However, we wish to argue that the approaches we have discussed so far provide an inadequate and partial account of the processes of case formulation. For example, cognitive models have been generated from laboratory studies in which subjects were asked to undertake problem-solving tasks involving both limited stimuli and limited choice. There is no such control in clinical encounters, where the clinician and client frequently confront each other as 'moving targets' struggling to comprehend each other's intentions (Cicourel 1999). In complex settings, the clinician's brain may just be much cleverer than the computer.

The relationship between the knower and the known

The abstracted rational–technical tools based on probability and utility depict the world of clinical practice as a peculiar, radically pared down, arid and emotionless space for the administration of clinical calculus. Cognitive, statistical and expert models all assume a stable clinical world out there waiting to be discovered. They fix this world as independent of the clinician and argue that it can become known only through objective and dispassionate inquiry and observation. This view of truth and knowledge is generally known in philosophy as **realism**, which

> presupposes a universal, homogeneous and essential human nature that allows knowers to be substituted for one another . . . Knowers are detached, neutral spectators, and the objects of knowledge are

separate from them, inert items in the observational knowledge-gathering process.

(Code 1995: 24–5)

We discuss this concept further in Chapter 2, but here we want to note that, in the context of clinical judgement, somewhat paradoxically, 'realism' of this kind is in many ways very *unrealistic*. We advocate that closer attention be paid to the social and cultural contexts in which professional judgements take place. 'Clinical decision-making is not the outcome of individual minds, operating in a social vacuum' (Atkinson 1995: 54). Like any other domain, it is subject to other influences. For example, decision-support models share the construction of 'the decision' as an event, arising either from an encounter of an individual clinician with a patient or from the competent use of a diagnostic formula like Bayes or an expert model. Sociological studies of clinical settings, however, have challenged this notion and illustrated how:

> In many organizational settings ... decision-making itself is a collective organizational activity ... 'decisions' may be subject to debate, negotiation and revision, based on talk within and between groups or teams of practitioners ... The silent inner dialogue of single-handed decision-making, therefore, is by no means the whole story.

(Atkinson 1995: 52)

If the individualist, information-processing models have their limits in biomedicine, then they appear even more impoverished when applied to domains of professional practice, such as therapeutics and social care, where negotiation, argument and persuasion are central to the processes of professional 'knowledge-making' (see, for example, Stancombe and White 1998; Ivey *et al.* 1999; Taylor and White 2000). Atkinson, above, stresses the importance of language, talk and context in the processes of judgement. This is a theme we develop in the rest of this chapter and throughout the book, where we explore competing social scientific ways of understanding clinical judgement. Our discussion follows three themes, all of which are developed at length in subsequent chapters of the book. These themes are:

- the historical, social and cultural nature of knowledge and the shifting repertoires of 'competent' professional understandings;
- the role of 'intuition' or 'practical wisdom' in clinical judgement;
- the importance of language, particularly storytelling and persuasion, in clinical judgement.

The artfulness of science and the science of artfulness

> On occasions when clinicians are in full possession of the necessary information, the hard scientific facts, they still must allow for their subjectivity, the fallibility of the tests' technology, and the uncontrollable variable that is the patient. Black polar bears, the bêtes noirs of inductive reasoning, prowl constantly through the thickets of medical knowledge: this patient may confound the rules, requiring the special exercise of clinical judgement, may even provoke the clinical insight that will eventuate in new knowledge.
>
> (Hunter 1991: 40)

Here, Hunter is pointing to the inevitable role of subjectivity in clinicians' use of 'objective' criteria to guide their judgements. In the statistical and cognitive approaches, subjectivity, in the shape of feelings, emotion or what may generically be termed 'intuition', is treated as a form of intellectual tinnitus – a persistent but essentially meaningless noise getting in the way of a good calculation. In contrast, for Hunter subjectivity and uncertainty are not contaminating forces to be neutralized, but inevitable, dynamic, essential parts of clinical judgement that merit investigation in their own right.

For example, as noted above, the 'facts' of a case rarely speak for themselves: to assess its relevance and its validity, even relatively 'hard' information derived from X-rays or laboratory tests requires interpretation. The 'facts' of a case are frequently approximations and equivocations, requiring the exercise of qualitative judgement. In Chapter 4, we consider an example from White's ethnographic study of paediatrics. The case concerns an eight-month-old baby, Joanne, who presented with an injury to her right leg. The paediatrician examining the child and her X-rays on admission was of the opinion that the leg was fractured. Moreover, unconvinced by the mother's account of the circumstances of the injury, he had raised concerns that the child might have sustained a non-accidental injury. Second opinions were sought from orthopaedic consultants and radiologists. Despite considering precisely the same X-rays, the different clinicians could reach no agreement about the nature and extent of the injury, or indeed about whether it was a fracture at all.

The paediatrician and other professionals involved in the case still had to act. They had to formulate their accounts of what happened to Joanne and their opinions about her future safety. Their responsibility did not end with diagnosis, although as we have said that was difficult enough in itself. They also had to ask 'who did it?', 'in what circumstances?' and 'will it happen again?' There were no algorithms to help them. They had to rely on other methods, such as their assessment of the plausibility of the mother's story, how she responded to the child and vice versa, and what they could find out about the family history. Thus, the 'science' of clinical practice, the generation of explanation from data, is itself artful, but of what does this artfulness consist and how may we open it up for investigation? For some, artfulness is simply artistry, or intuition.

Tacit knowledge: is intuition enough?

> From the perspective of Technical Rationality, professional practice is a process of problem *solving*. Problems of choice or decision are solved through the selection, from available means, of the one best suited to established ends. But with this emphasis on problem solving, we ignore problem *setting*, the process by which we define the decision to be made, the ends to be achieved, the means which may be chosen. In real world practice, problems do not present themselves to the practitioner as givens. They must be constructed from the materials of problematic situations which are puzzling, troubling and uncertain.
>
> (Schön 1988: 65–6)

Like Hunter, Donald Schön sees uncertainty as inevitable in professional practice. He accepts that some problems can be solved by the application of the artefacts of science, in the form of research-based theory and technique. This is the 'high hard ground' of practice (Schön 1988: 67), but the problems that can be addressed on this firm terrain are the most straightforward, such as 'is this a case of chicken pox?' For Schön, the most important professional questions arise in the 'swampy lowlands' (Schön 1988: 67), and here practitioners must rely not on external knowledge provided by theory or science, but on something within themselves, some form of artistry, craft or intuition. Drawing on Polanyi's (1967) concept of **tacit knowledge** (knowledge that we have but take for granted and find difficult to articulate), Schön constructs the competent clinician as a spontaneous and skilful *actor*, who just 'knows' how to act. This actor becomes aware of using particular knowledge and skills only at certain times:

> Much reflection in action hinges on the element of surprise. When intuitive, spontaneous performance yields nothing more than the results expected for it, then we tend not to think about it. But when intuitive performance leads to surprises, pleasing and promising or unwanted, we may respond by reflecting-in-action.
>
> (Schön 1988: 72)

Reflection-*in*-action is different from reflection-*on*-action, since it is embedded in the action-present. It is contained *in* the action at a point where it will make a difference. Schön's work has been very influential in those occupations operating in the 'swampy lowlands', such as therapy, social work and nursing.

For example, Benner and her colleagues (Benner 1987; Benner *et al.* 1996) have undertaken a number of studies examining nurses' clinical reasoning and decision-making as practical expertise or 'know-how'. The development of 'know-how' depends on mastery over time of the many variables that nurses confront in clinical practice. While there are some echoes of the cognitive approach, the focus on nurses' 'know-how' in Benner's studies is similar to Schön's concept of knowledge-in-action. Nurses become 'expert' when they have an *intuitive* grasp of what to do and can function without consulting formal rules and procedural guidance. This intuitive knowledge draws upon and incorporates formal knowledge, but not necessarily in a self-conscious way.

Where the cognitive scientists and statisticians are pessimistic about human reasoning, for Schön hope springs eternal. He is optimistic and trusting about the intuitive reasoning processes of professionals (Dowie and Elstein 1988). One has to hope that his trust is well placed, since his model gives few clues as to how the tacit dimension may be investigated. For example, Schön fails adequately to develop his ideas about reflection-*on*-action. But without the 'distance' created by the rigorous analysis of *past* interventions, it is difficult to see how the clinician could develop the critical capacity for reflection-*in*-action. Tacit knowledge has the potential to make us very confident about our competence as practitioners, but it may also lead to uncritical practice where we simply assert that X or Y is true because 'we just know it'. Rolfe (1998) is critical of Benner's work on these grounds. He cites the following example to indicate the dangers of 'just knowing'. 'When I say to a doctor "the patient is psychotic", I don't know always how to legitimate the statement, but I am never wrong. Because I know psychosis inside out. And I feel that, and I know it and I trust it' (Benner 1984, cited in Rolfe 1998: 51). Taylor and White (2000: 193) note:

> This is a good illustration of the difficulties that intuitive practice may produce. We have probably all felt at some time or other that 'we can't explain it, we just know' and sometimes we will have been right. But we do get into difficulties with 'just knowing' especially when 'we are never wrong'. This inaccessibility of our judgements is very problematic since we cannot share the basis of them with other people ... If we are to have dialogue with other professionals and with clients then we need to be able to articulate the basis for our judgements.
>
> (Taylor and White 2000: 193)

What Hunter refers to as 'black polar bears', threatening the execution of 'objective' clinical reasoning, do not come disguised only as recalcitrant patients and inconclusive test results. They also come in the much stealthier form of tacit presuppositions and preferred formulations, camouflaged against the familiar thickets of our professional imagination. To pick out these bears, and decide whether or not they bite, we need something to help us interrogate 'intuition'. We need a 'science' (of sorts) of artfulness.

The need to develop technologies to aid reflection-on-action has been recognized in the professional literature. However, the proposed models have tended to reduce reflection to a process of 'benign introspection' (Woolgar 1988: 22). The practitioner is urged to look *inward*, to reflect, for example, upon how their own life experiences or significant events may have impacted upon their thinking, or how their feelings about the patient/client may have led to biases or professional failings. Typically, this form of reflection involves the practitioner keeping confessional diaries, which include critical accounts of their actions 'in the field'. The following typical example is taken from nursing and has been analysed in greater detail (by Carolyn Taylor) in Taylor and White (2000: 195):

> I believe I was guilty of causing Peter harm in this way by sometimes bowing to pressure from his relatives and partner. If I were to do anything different it would have to be to remember I am accountable and responsible for my patient; I must always put them first.
>
> In being involved in the situation, by being aware of the components of the situation and then by examining my responses, I believe I have become increasingly more effective in my work by the knowledge gained through reflective practice.
>
> (Graham 1998: 130–1)

This account does nothing to interrogate the tacit assumptions and presuppositions of contemporary nursing practice. Instead, it simply reproduces them in another form. Moreover, by confining her misdemeanours and errors to the *past* and displaying her capacity to learn from her mistakes, the nurse constructs her *current* practice as new, improved, more competent and less open to challenge. Through their confessionals, clinicians often cast themselves as born-again truth brokers. This effectively closes down challenge and debate about their practice – the very thing reflective diaries are supposed to encourage.

> By introducing subjectivity, reflective writing brings us much closer to practice than objectivist accounts. But we also need to recognize that such accounts are not what 'really happened'. They are narrative accounts written up later and from one particular perspective. Often

they are written for a third party, such as a practice teacher or mentor, and to a particular format. They may be intended to demonstrate the writer's competence as a reflective practitioner as much as to develop specific areas of practice.

(Taylor and White 2000: 196)

So reflective diaries rely on particular use of language and have a social context. This context is not investigated in its own right, but it remains 'tacit', taken for granted and immune from analysis (Rolfe 1998; Ixer 1999; Taylor and White 2000). A proper investigation of context would involve looking not just *inwards* to our personal flaws and biases, but *outwards* to the social and cultural artefacts and forms of thought that constitute what we currently think of as competent professional judgement. Thus, we would need to be able to interrogate our favoured professional stories to defamiliarize our tacit knowledge. For help with this, we must turn to the humanities (Little 1995; Downie and Macnaughton 2000) and social sciences.

Storytelling and persuasion in case formulation

Professionals are involved in acts of meaning-making, which are often collaborative and are bound by available repertoires of interpretation. Meaning-making is accomplished through language and takes place in particular social and organizational contexts. In order to get their job done, professionals must package their opinions for consumption by others. They must be able to justify, account for and 'perform' their judgements. This may be for the patient or client who has come to their service, or for colleagues, or in some other arena of accountability or judgement-making, like the courts or a clinical audit. They must also 'work up' a written account of aspects of their thinking for case files, reports and records.

Moreover, patients/clients come to services with their own stories to tell. So the processes of clinical judgement are intrinsically 'storied'. Professionals 'take the history', then retell it in a form consistent with their specialist knowledge. However, professional **narratives** contain more than specialist knowledge. They attribute cause and effect and often construct blameworthiness and creditworthiness. Professional stories, even humorous anecdotes, are often moral tales. This is something we consider at length elsewhere in this book.

It is easy for the notion of 'storytelling' to be misunderstood. We are not suggesting that the patient's body, the family's problems or the child's injury do not exist outside of the story. Instead, 'troubles' are given particular meanings, which may, for example, construct them as the proper business of the professional, or alternatively as the proper business of another. It is worthwhile at this point to say a little more about our particular use of the concepts of narrative and storytelling. Mishler (1986) defines narrative as a particular kind of 'recapitulation' that preserves 'the temporal ordering of events' and presents those events as the antecedents or consequences of each other. That is, narratives embody a 'consequential sequencing: one event causes another' (Reissman 1993: 17). So narratives attribute cause and effect in particular ways. These aspects of stories Edwards calls 'the occasioned, action-performative workings of discourse' (Edwards 1997: 276). By this he refers to the *work* stories perform in social contexts. We want to argue that these action-performative or **rhetorical** features of professional stories have particular importance for understanding clinical judgement.

When we talk of 'rhetoric' or 'rhetorical potency', we are referring simply to 'powerful talk' (Potter and Wetherell 1995: 82). Used in this way, rhetoric does not imply deceitfulness. Nor is a 'rhetorical' utterance empty of facts (Billig *et al.* 1988), as is sometimes implied, for example, when journalists refer to 'political rhetoric'. Instead, we are referring to words and phrases that do a particular job of persuading, by mobilizing facts in a specific order, with certain emphases, usually drawing on culturally dominant ideas. It will be helpful if we illustrate our point with an example from professional practice.

Extract 1.1
Con: Ben Owen – you've not had the pleasure, of this mother. Mother is under our psychiatrists she is a (2.0) oh (2.0) factitious illness gives the wrong impression. She's got a [neurotic] state really, somatization
Reg: [Right] right
Con: [Somatization], really *severe* somatization disorder
Reg: [Right] yeah
Con: You, you may have met her [. . . as soon as you meet her, she'll go on] – he's CONstipated, severely CONstipated
Reg: [I think I probably, what's he got?] Yes, it's all, yes
Con: She looks ill and as soon as you meet her she looks ill and she'll come out with all of her complaints. He has severe CONstipation actually required a ( ) when they first brought him in to extract the masses of faeces, but recently he's relapsed and the problem seemed to be that mum had relapsed as well so everything went (.) down and he had to come in for an enema –
Reg: That's right, that's right. That's how I know him, I didn't [see him]
Con: [No well] and mum couldn't er, it had to be done here cos mum can't cope at home, she can't cope. He was much better, but he was on sort of 30 mls of Picolax a day. His bowel is just sort of –
Reg: – Huge

This extract is taken from a discussion between a consultant paediatrician and a registrar at the beginning of a paediatric outpatient clinic. The consultant begins by stating the child's name, 'Ben Owen'. However, the 'mother' is immediately introduced as a troublesome party with the ironic statement 'you've not had the pleasure' and by assigning her to the deviant category 'psychiatric patient'. With the statement, 'You, you may have met her [. . . as soon as you meet her, she'll go on] – he's constipated, severely constipated', the consultant makes an implicit link between the symptom (constipation) and the mother's character. This needs very little elaboration; its relevance is not questioned by the registrar, who appears to hear it as an account of what caused the problem. That is, by describing the mother and her behaviour, the consultant establishes the child's complaint as a psychological response to inappropriate parental management (for example, 'recently he's relapsed and the problem seemed to be that mum had relapsed as well' and 'mum couldn't er, it had to be done here cos mum can't cope at home, she can't cope'). Moreover, the consultant's experience of hearing the mother's 'illness stories' has had a clear effect on her opinion of what caused the problem. Of course, it is also based on physical palpation of the abdomen and on specialist knowledge (for example, that 'chronic idiopathic constipation of childhood' often has a psychological component), but these are only part of a much richer repertoire of meaning-making processes. These different 'rationalities' (for example, science, experience, professional intuition) tend not to be arranged hierarchically on a scale from more to less reliable, but are treated as equally valid (Atkinson 1995).

If clinicians rely on a range of different kinds of knowledge and warrants in their judgement-making, we need to recognize these and explore them as topics in their own right. This requires us to suspend judgement about the adequacy of clinicians' judgements and examine instead how judgements get done in the cut and thrust of everyday clinical activity. In Part 2 of this book we do just this, but first we must explore in more detail some of the assumptions and presuppositions that have affected contemporary understandings of professional judgement (Chapter 2) and what forms of inquiry and reasoning are excluded by them (Chapter 3).

Summary

- Approaches to clinical judgement are generally concerned with two analytically separable questions: '*how* clinicians make judgements and decisions and *how well* they make them' (Dowie and Elstein 1988: 2). The vast majority of work in the field is concerned with the second question. It is normative and evaluative, concerned with uncovering error and improving consistency.

- Approaches differ in their treatment of the concept of uncertainty. There is some agreement that uncertainty exists in clinical activity and may cause problems for clinicians, but there is considerable disagreement about its inevitability, and its tractability.
- Clinical judgements may be seen primarily as internal, cognitive actions undertaken by the practitioner, who is seen as an independent, thinking entity. Alternatively, they may be seen as products (at least in part) of social processes, such as the circulation and reproduction of dominant ideas (or discourses) about the right and proper way to classify and treat particular problems at specific times. We have argued that both these ways of thinking about professional judgement are important, but in the contemporary policy climate, the former has become privileged and has eclipsed the latter.
- Approaches differ in the extent to which they assume a fixed and stable world out there waiting to be discovered. Realist models assume a stable knowledge base, independent of the professional and the institutional context in which they are working. Other models stress the capacity of language to construct the way we see the real world. Knowledge is seen as a product of historical and social processes. This is not the same as saying that reality does not exist, but it raises questions about how we make sense of and order that reality through our talk, our stories and our preferred formulations.
- The old adage that clinical judgement is both an art and a science still dominates much of the literature, along with concerns about the types of reasoning processes clinicians (should) use. These debates typically raise questions such as: What is the role of intuition and how does this differ from analytical thinking? Can clinicians be trusted to be intuitive? Is the clinician best characterized as a scientist, or as a detective, or as a moral judge? How do ('cold') technical processes interact with ('warm') humane judgements?
- We have sought to 'trouble' the art–science, head–heart distinctions and to argue that the practice of science requires artfulness, while the processes involved in artfulness and intuition require analysis in their own right.

2 Seductive certainties
The 'scientific-bureaucratic' model

Chapter 1 outlined the various ways in which the processes of clinical judgement have been understood. There are statistical models, based on the assumption that uncertainty is tractable, that neutral facts are the constituent elements of judgement-making and that the correct interpretation of the case results from inserting these facts into appropriate statistical formulae. In these models, the clinician's brain is seen as a flawed instrument for the collection and interpretation of facts. Objective reasoning is valued above all else, while subjectivity is seen as a murky contaminant to proper judgement-making. In this model, the crafting of a case formulation is analogous to a draughtsman's drawing. It relies on skill, knowledge and technique, but it differs from 'art' because it is uncontaminated by imagination and emotion. In contrast, other models stress the importance of experience and seasoned professional intuition. The clinician's subjectivity becomes a positive force, and the act of judgement-making a form of artistry, a magnificent freehand flourish created using the medium of formal knowledge, but not reducible to it. We concluded the chapter by arguing that, while these optimistic intuitive models appear to accept the complexity involved in clinical encounters, they offer no adequate means by which clinicians' 'tacit knowledge' may be investigated. Intuition runs unchecked. We argued that professional stories, which draw on common sense, emotion and formal knowledge in artful ways, are central components of clinical judgement and demand rigorous exploration in their own right.

In making their judgements, professionals make use of a number of different kinds of reasoning, all of which are important for understanding the processes of case formulation. However, these different ways of knowing are not equally acknowledged and represented in policy developments and practice guidance. In this chapter, we show that one particular form of rationality underpins contemporary policy initiatives such as New Labour's modernization programme in the UK. This rationality, termed by Harrison (1999) the 'scientific-bureaucratic' model, is currently influencing policy and practice across the range of health and welfare professions.

Harrison (1999: 3) defines the 'scientific-bureaucratic' model as follows:

> Scientific-bureaucratic [rationality] . . . centres on the assumption
> that valid and reliable knowledge is mainly to be obtained from the
> accumulation of research conducted by experts according to strict
> scientific criteria . . . It further assumes that working clinicians are
> likely to be both too busy and insufficiently skilled to interpret
> and apply such knowledge for themselves, and therefore holds that
> professional practice should be influenced through the systematic
> aggregation by academic experts of research findings on a particular
> topic, and the distillation of such findings into protocols and
> guidelines which may then be communicated to practitioners with
> the expectation that practice will be improved . . . The logic, though
> not always the overt form, of guidelines is essentially algorithmic.

So this model is 'scientific' in the sense that it promises a secure knowledge
base that can provide rational foundations for clinical decisions. It is bureaucratic in the sense that this knowledge is codified and manualized through the
use of protocols, guidelines and computer models, adherence to which may be
monitored by managers or through internal and external audit.

Scientific-bureaucratic rationality has found its pinnacle in the evidence-
based practice (EBP) movement, which, as we have noted, has now achieved
the status of official policy in the NHS in the UK and in the USA. On one
level, this policy is sensible and uncontroversial. It is wholly proper that professionals should pay attention to 'what works' when they prescribe drugs or
plan other interventions, and therefore they need reliable data on just these
kinds of issues. Moreover, the series of high-profile professional scandals that
have hit the UK press in recent years appear to support the view that clinicians
can no longer be assumed to be authoritative experts in a given sphere of
competence, but may be sources of (occasionally deadly) error or malevolence.
These scandals include the actions of Harold Shipman, a GP who murdered
several of his patients (2000), the perioperative deaths of babies due to the
incompetence of surgeons at the Bristol Royal Infirmary during the 1990s, the
removal of organs without consent at Alder Hey Children's Hospital (2001)
and failures on the part of child welfare agencies to protect children at risk,
exemplified by the death of Victoria Climbié (2001). As a response to these
events and others like them, calls for greater bureaucratization, systematiza-
tion and control have a common-sense appeal.

However, we want to argue here that while attempts to bureaucratize,
audit and control practice may be *necessary* components of any attempt to
regulate professionals and to prevent error and abuse, they are not on their
own *sufficient*. Moreover, they can have unintended consequences and may
sometimes provide a poor fit with the realities of professional practice in

many settings. In order to understand the near monopoly that rational-technical forms of governance appear to have attained, we must look more carefully at their antecedents. For this we must first examine the policy developments and organizational changes that have taken place over the past two decades, and then locate these changes more broadly in relation to ideas about truth and knowledge.

Political pragmatism: the ascent of scientific-bureaucratic rationality

It may be argued that the historical conditions that facilitated the ascent of EBP were not as much the desire to correct error as an attempt to control resources. That is, EBP provides a handy rationale to accomplish a shift from implicit to explicit rationing of health care (Harrison 1998). For example, it is clear that during the 1980s the Conservative government of the time was under considerable pressure to contain costs. One mechanism for so doing was to limit the freedom of doctors to prescribe and treat: hence the introduction of the technologies of general management, such as delegated budgets, 'cost improvements' and clinical audit. In 1991, the NHS Research and Development (R & D) initiative was established specifically to evaluate the efficacy of certain treatments and ensure cost-effectiveness. During the 1990s, the introduction of quasi-market principles and the separation of purchaser and provider services institutionalized the rationing function (Harrison 1998: 19). The decisions of health authorities were based on questions of cost-efficiency, effectiveness and quality of service (Flynn and Williams 1997; Ham, 1999), with some of their decisions proving controversial, such as the case of Jaymee Bowen (child B), who was denied a further bone marrow transplant to treat her leukaemia because the odds of a positive outcome were considered to be unacceptably low (see New 1996). These technologies eroded certain aspects of medical autonomy as it had been traditionally understood (Flynn 1992; Harrison and Pollitt 1994; Harrison and Ahmed 2000).

In 1997, the freshly elected 'New Labour' government announced its intention to remove the more competitive elements of the quasi-market, and health authorities, trusts and GPs were encouraged to cooperate and collaborate in the interests of patients and communities (Department of Health 1997). However, it seems clear that the new government somewhat overstated the divisive and competitive aspects of the quasi-market as it worked in practice (Flynn and Williams 997). Thus, despite the rhetoric of change and reform and the promise of increased investment, New Labour's health policy is characterized more by continuity than by revolution. While the discourse of quality and consumerism may have superseded the language of the market in health and social care agencies, the concern with increasing efficiency and cost-effectiveness remains. Moreover, the understandable public concern about incompetent or maleficent professionals has ensured that bureaucratization and control remain firmly on the policy agenda. It is the concepts and methods associated with EBP that are seen to hold the promise for dealing with each of these pressing 'quality', 'control' and 'cost-effectiveness' imperatives.

Thus, EBP is now the cornerstone of NHS policy in the UK and is equally dominant in the USA, where the insurance companies are naturally keen to avoid spending money on ineffective treatments. In the UK, New Labour has introduced a number of initiatives to ensure the implementation of evidence-based approaches, including the framework known as clinical governance: 'through which NHS organisations are accountable for continuously improving the quality of their services and safeguarding high standards of care by creating an environment in which excellence in clinical care will flourish' (NHS Executive 1998: 33). Clinical governance is an umbrella term encompassing a range of audit, risk management and quality assurance activities that are now built into the day-to-day business in health care provider agencies. Managers and practitioners in services are given joint responsibility for the quality of services and the development of best practice based on 'sound evidence' disseminated in guidelines and protocols.

This internal auditing activity has been augmented by the establishment in 1999 of two new bodies, the National Institute for Clinical Excellence (NICE) and the Commission for Health Improvement (CHI). The former has the role of undertaking 20–30 appraisals of new interventions each year, which are intended to inform a range of clinical guidelines or protocols that clinicians are expected to follow (unless they can make a very good case against so doing). CHI is a body quasi-independent from government and one of its functions will be to monitor the compliance of services with the guidelines issued by NICE.

There have been similar developments in social care, with the establishment in 2001 of the General Social Care Council, which has a range of regulatory functions in the social care sector and the Social Care Institute for Excellence (SCIE). The rationale for this body is almost identical to that of NICE. SCIE is described in a Department of Health press release as follows:

> SCIE will create a knowledge base of what works in social care and the information will be made available to managers, practitioners and users. It will rigorously review research and practice to provide a database of information on methods proven to be effective in social care practice. Using this information, SCIE will produce guidelines on Best Practice . . . The guidelines will also feed into the standards set by the Social Services Inspectorate, and ultimately those produced by the General Social Care Council and the National Care Standards

Commission, to monitor performance. This will mean users can then be confident that the services they receive have been tested against the best and most up-to-date knowledge in social care.

(Department of Health 2001a)

Self-evidently, EBP requires the accumulation of a substantial body of evidence upon which to base clinical decisions, which began in earnest in the UK with the establishment of the R & D programme in the 1990s. However, the evidence so generated is of a particular sort, focusing specifically on the effectiveness, or otherwise, of a range of interventions. As a source of such evidence, the randomized controlled trial (RCT) has become constructed as the *sine qua non* of medical research. That is to say, evidence-based practice has a clear 'hierarchy of evidence' (Canadian Task Force 1979), with RCTs at the top ostensibly providing a 'gold standard' against which all else can be judged. This would also appear to be the prescription for social care, as Gomm (2000: 51) asserts: 'The properly conducted, correctly interpreted RCT (randomised controlled trial) is superior to any other method for producing evidence about cause and effect. This includes evidence about the effectiveness of health and social care interventions.'

RCTs randomly allocate patients between a group who will receive the treatment under investigation and a control group who will receive a placebo (or no treatment) and/or an existing conventional treatment; ideally, neither the clinician nor the patient should know who is receiving the treatment (that is, the trial should be 'double-blind'). Meta-analyses and systematic reviews of RCTs are at the very pinnacle of the hierarchy of evidence. A range of specialist centres such as the Cochrane Centre in Oxford (named after Professor A. L. Cochrane, who, during the early 1970s, argued for and eventually popularized the RCT) have been established to scrutinize research findings for evidence of bias or other flaws in design. In social care, RCTs are rather more difficult to apply, but the concern with 'what works', which forms the mandate for the SCIE, will inevitably encourage research into population outcomes intended to inform action in individual cases.

What is wrong with evidence-based practice?

The simple answer to this question is of course 'nothing'. As we have noted, there is clearly an intrinsic correctness to the idea that professionals should not inflict upon patients or clients interventions that are ineffective or harmful, and it is self-evident that not all practitioners can be trusted to police themselves. However, we argue below that there are some problems with reducing the processes of clinical judgement to the question 'what works?' These are as follows:

1   The focus on treatment and outcome brackets out or over-simplifies the processes of case formulation, which must always precede decisions about interventions. These processes are complex and cannot be objectified or adequately represented in guidelines.

2   In its current form, EBP does not translate straightforwardly to some areas of professional practice, particularly those concerned with human relationships rather than with manipulating biological processes. However, there is evidence of a rather troubling colonization of these domains by scientific-bureaucratic rationality.

We consider these in turn.

Case formulation and EBP

> Evidence-based medicine is not 'cook-book' medicine. Because it requires a bottom-up approach that integrates the best external evidence with individual clinical expertise and patient choice, it cannot result in slavish cook-book approaches to individual patient care. External clinical evidence can inform, but can never replace, individual clinical expertise and it is this expertise that decides whether external evidence applies to the individual patient at all and, if so, how it should be integrated into a clinical decision . . . Clinicians who fear top-down cook-books will find the advocates of evidence-based medicine joining them at the barricades.
>
> (Sackett *et al.* 1997: 4)

Taken from one of the main texts on evidence-based medicine, the quotation above underscores the importance of clinicians' individual judgements and argues against the production of prescriptive recipes for particular interventions. It stresses that evidence from RCTs, based as it is on probabilities within particular populations, may not apply to individual patients, and thus the clinician must exercise careful judgement. Yet, as we have seen, in its current incarnation as the cornerstone of health service policy, it is precisely as cook-book knowledge that evidence-based practice appears to be being prescribed. Moreover, RCTs are unconcerned with the causation of disease, distress or cure. They are not trying to establish why a treatment works, or to uncover the mysteries of causation. They concentrate solely on establishing correlations between treatments and outcomes (Harrison 1998; Downie and Macnaughton 2000). This is a radically different form of knowledge from that generated by traditional biomedical research, which is centrally concerned with establishing 'what's wrong?'; that is, with elucidating the normal and pathological workings of the body.

We suggest that the question 'what's wrong?' is also the central concern in most clinical encounters. Whether they are concerned with biology or human relationships, clinicians are trying to formulate a story about what might be going on. Without this story, they cannot proceed to treatment and outcome and they cannot decide whether the population probabilities generated by RCTs apply to this particular patient, at this particular time, attending this particular service. Moreover, case formulation often involves moral and emotional judgements, about, for example, whether a particular individual could cope with a demanding treatment regimen, or whether a parent is telling the truth about their child's suspicious injury. In these circumstances, an outcome-oriented evidence base is frankly neither use nor ornament.

So EBP assumes a great deal about the ways in which clinicians make sense of cases. In their rush to decide what *ought* to happen, policy-makers have forgotten to examine what *is* happening in real encounters. Yet, as we noted in Chapter 1, there is a substantial literature from, for example, within medical sociology to show that in producing formulations for the cases they confront, clinicians rely on a range of warrants for their opinions, with personal anecdotes, appeals to 'common sense', professional identity and moral judgement playing their part. We examine some of these studies in detail in Part 2, but our argument here is that these kinds of reasoning cannot simply be bracketed out, or treated as sources of bias or error. They are important ways of understanding the clinical encounter in all its social complexity. In the context of case formulation, the 'evidence base' is but one form of knowledge. For other types of judgement, we need different ways of knowing, but these kinds of thinking and understanding are being sidelined, marginalized or even ridiculed by certain proponents of EBP. We are thus in danger of being left without a vocabulary with which to think about or debate the realities of professional practice.

Colonizing care: an example

We have already suggested that in most, if not all, clinical settings the pared down version of professional judgement constructed by EBP (as it is currently understood) is in many ways unrealistic. It is not how professionals do business, and with the exception of certain discrete areas of activity (for example, 'Do I prescribe drug a or b?'; 'Will surgery or chemotherapy be most effective?') it never could be. Showing the folly of the assumption that all aspects of clinical judgement can be objictified in this way is the purpose of this book, and we have a good deal more to say about it in subsequent chapters. However, the assumptions of EBP and the reign of the RCT have become inextricably tied up with legitimation of professional activity and the allocation of resources – so much so that areas of activity such as therapeutics and social care have become steadily colonized and the interventions associated with these types of care treated as though they are analogous to the treatment regimens of biomedicine. This is despite the fact that, beyond the evaluation of cognitive–behavioural programmes of various kinds (Sheldon 1999; Sheldon and MacDonald 1999), experimental designs have not proved very successful: 'Even in the US, where empirical social work is at its most advanced, the outcomes of experimental and quasi-experimental studies have yielded comparatively little fruit' (Trinder 2000: 150).

Psychotherapy process research provides a particularly interesting example of the colonization to which we have referred and it is worth examining in more detail (for more complex analyses of the methodological debates see Stancombe and White 1998; Owen 1999). Since the time of Breuer and Freud, psychotherapy has been formulated in one form or another as the 'talking cure', and this assumption has long underpinned the research programme for psychotherapy:

> The patient communicates something; the therapist communicates something in response; the patient communicates and/or experiences something different; and the therapist, patient and others like the change. What the therapist communicates (the independent variables) is very likely multidimensional (and the pattern of the multidimensionality needs to be specified) and may be different at different phases of the interaction for different kinds of patients. Similarly, what the patient communicates and/or experiences differently (the dependent variables) is likely multidimensional (and the pattern of the multidimensionality needs to be clarified) and may be different at distinct phases of the interaction. The enormous task of psychotherapy theory and research is that of filling in the variables of this paradigm.
>
> (Kiesler 1966: 130)

This paradigm has become known as the 'drug metaphor' (Stiles and Shapiro 1989), as it clearly draws explicit analogies between psychotherapy and psychopharmacological research. That is, the paradigm views psychotherapy as comprising 'active ingredients' (for example, interpretations, confrontation, reflection), which are supplied by the therapist to the client, along with a variety of 'fillers' and scene-setting features. At the most simplistic level, if a component is 'active' then 'high levels' within therapy should predict more positive outcomes. If this is not the case then the 'ingredient' is assumed to be 'inert'.

Clearly, the drug metaphor in psychotherapy process research precedes the evidence-based practice movement by some three decades, and owes some of its dominance to the medical lineage of psychotherapy. However, its significance has been amplified by the demands of the scientific bureaucratic rationality and in particular the requirements of clinical governance. This is despite a growing critique of the paradigm from within psychotherapy process research and the persistent failure of these methods to undercover the basic mechanisms of therapeutic change. In particular, the drug metaphor has been criticized on the following grounds:

1   It assumes that process and outcome are readily distinguishable from each other; that is, that client outcomes are a direct linear product of therapeutic process. In pharmaceutical trials, drugs can be manipulated independently of the patient's condition, but in psychotherapy, process components may reflect changes or 'outcomes' that have already occurred, or are the result of some life event not directly related to the therapy.

2   It makes assumptions about 'dosage'; that is, that 'active' ingredients of specific therapies remain constant, regardless of who is practising the therapy and their relationship with the patient, an assumption that Stiles and Shapiro (1989: 527) deem 'absurd'.

3   Despite the very real differences that exist between various kinds of therapy in relation to theoretical orientation, techniques and interviewing practices, the outcomes for patients appear to be very similar. This 'equivalence paradox' (Stiles *et al.* 1986) again calls into question the notion of linear change based on a number of variables which can somehow be isolated from the therapeutic relationship.

4   The drug metaphor ignores the effects of the communicative practices of the client (Stiles and Shapiro 1989). Clients are not inert. They make contingent choices about what they introduce as a topic for discussion, what they conceal and what they reveal, as Owen (1999: 205) notes: 'Rather than all therapeutic input lying under the control of the therapist, it is also the case that clients and their abilities play a part in regulating therapy and in becoming "active ingredients" in making their own changes.'

However, despite this trenchant criticism, the drug metaphor is still alive and dominant within contemporary reviews of psychotherapy process research (Kaye 1995; Stancombe and White 1998; Owen 1999), as Kaye notes:

> The relative failure of psychotherapy research to either establish the variables contributing to psychotherapeutic change or to put psychotherapy on a scientific footing has provoked little questioning of the assumptive base of this research. It has led rather to a consistent effort to refine experimental design and methodology.
>
> (Kaye 1995: 38)

Thus, despite the problems in the use of RCTs in psychotherapy, they remain the gold standard at the top of the hierarchy of evidence (Parry and Richardson 1996; Department of Health 2001b).

We are not making any claims one way or another about the effectiveness of psychotherapy. We are simply arguing that the drug metaphor is seriously misplaced. So why is it that researchers persist in paring down an activity so bound up in the communicative practices of therapist and client, and so self-evidently laden with contingent social meanings and matters of relationship and trust, to a set of 'ingredients', ostensibly separable from their medium of transmission? The answer to this is complex and clearly relates in part to the discussion earlier in this chapter about rationing and resource constraints. Under the current policy regime 'demonstrating effectiveness' has become essential to securing and sustaining funding. In many senses, as we have already noted, this is perfectly right and proper, but clinical activity is not reducible to outcome and neither can process and outcome be clearly separated in all cases. The demands of policy are producing a version of clinical judgement that cannot in reality exist. In order to understand why the particular form of 'knowing' associated with objectivity and statistical models has become so dominant we must go back further into the history of thought and explore the way in which knowledge and truth have come to be understood. For this, we must leave behind contemporary policy and research agendas and examine the effects of a particularly robust cultural narrative, which influences all aspects of our lives. In order to understand what is being assumed by EPB, we need to visit one of its elderly and particularly influential relatives: the seventeenth-century philosophy of the **Enlightenment**.

The Enlightenment: reason, progress and science

The 'Enlightenment' is a Western European philosophical movement, principally associated with the work of French philosopher Descartes. The Enlightenment marks the dawn of the age of reason, or **modernity** in Western Europe, and the ideas associated with it course through our contemporary understandings of knowledge, truth, reason and rationality. These ideas have become so dominant that, outside philosophy and the social sciences, they are generally taken for granted and treated as the only right and proper way to think. The main themes of Enlightenment thought can be summarized as follows:

> First, a concept of freedom based upon an autonomous human subject who is capable of acting in a conscious manner. Second, the pursuit of a universal and foundational 'truth' gained through a correspondence of ideas with social and physical reality. Third, a

belief in the natural sciences as the correct model for thinking about the social and natural world over, for example, theology and metaphysics. Fourth, the accumulation of systematic knowledge with the progressive unfolding of history.

(May 1996: 8)

Modernity, then, is associated with the steady march of reason and progress and the cumulative nature of knowledge. Once created, using the techniques of scientific inquiry, knowledge is seen to reproduce the real world and hence can be used again and again by any number of inquirers, providing they are able to separate their messy emotions from their reasoning. Quantification soon assumed particular importance in this new form of knowledge, as it allowed for standardization over space and time and seemed to offer certainty in place of contingent personal judgement: 'The pre-industrial world privileged personal judgement over objectivity. By contrast, the modern world privileges objectivity, the withdrawal of human agency and its replacement by impartial uniformity' (Dahlberg *et al.* 1999: 88). The influence of this thinking on contemporary policy is self-evident and it is easy for us to forget that there are any other ways of understanding knowledge, truth and judgement.

Shaking the certainty

The Enlightenment version of objectivity relies on the separation of the capacity for reason (performed by a disciplined brain or, even better, by a computer simulation of a disciplined brain) from a feeling, emoting 'body', and from other minds, and from language and history. We can clearly see the influence of these ideas about knowledge and reason in some of the approaches to clinical judgement discussed in Chapter 1.

The sociologist of science Bruno Latour (1999) uses the metaphor 'brain-in-a-vat' to describe the enduring and pervasive legacy of this separation of mind and body. For Latour, this particular 'take' on knowledge and truth causes distortions in the way we see the world: 'Inhuman, reductionist, causal, law-like, objective, cold, unanimous, absolute – all these expressions do not pertain to nature *as such*, but to nature viewed through the deforming prism of the glass vessel' (Latour 1999: 10). This is a similar point to one we made above in relation to psychotherapy process research. In an attempt to legitimate its activity and prove its efficacy, process researchers have constructed a version of therapy as reductionist, causal and law-like, but this does not fit with therapy in real time. Latour argues that there are other ways of understanding the relationship between what exists and how we know it, but these understandings require us to follow pathways that have become increasingly overgrown by the Enlightenment version of realism, at the heart of which Latour sees a troubling paradox:

> Why in the first place did we need the idea of an *outside world* looked at through a gaze from the very uncomfortable observation post of a mind-in-a-vat? ... And why burden this solitary mind with the impossible task of finding absolute certainty instead of plugging it into the connections that would provide it with all the relative certainties it needed to know and to act? Why shout out of both sides of our mouths these two contradictory orders 'Be absolutely disconnected!' 'Find absolute proof that you are connected!' Who could untangle such a double bind?
>
> (Latour 1999: 12)

Latour is arguing that the form of realism constructed in Enlightenment thought is only one of a number of ways of understanding the nature of knowledge (known in philosophy as **epistemology**). However, his rhetorical question at the start of the quote is a serious one, which merits attention. The reason why we cling so desperately to the idea of uncontaminated objective truth is the fear that, if we give up on it, we may open the door to an 'anything goes' philosophical position, where all beliefs are purely subjective and therefore equal. Under such conditions, for example, the actions of Harold Shipman could be justified on the grounds that killing his patients made him happy, the failures of Bristol surgeons on the grounds that they felt they needed the practice, the removal of organs without consent on the grounds that the children no longer needed them or the murder of Victoria Climbié because she really was possessed by the devil.

These kinds of worries are often raised in relation to a philosophical position known as **relativism**. This is closely associated with **social constructionism** (see Taylor and White 2000 for a more detailed discussion of this concept in relation to health and welfare practice), which rejects the idea that we can totally disconnect ourselves from the world in order to study it and argues that language inevitably also constructs what it seeks to describe. So these positions stress the historical and contingent nature of knowledge and reject the idea of absolute and final versions. This makes people uncomfortable for all the reasons we have given above. However, it is only worrying if we cling to the idea that the rigours of natural science are the only legitimate ways of knowing anything. We argue below that this is not the case. There are ways of knowing and judging that are not, and indeed cannot be, based on algorithms because none exist, but this does not mean we cannot act and nor does it mean that we are incapable of deciding between good and bad ideas. However, for the relativists, the question of judgement is much more contingent, it depends on the circumstances, as Knorr-Cetina and Mulkay (1983: 6) note:

The belief that scientific knowledge does not merely replicate nature *in no way* commits the epistemic relativist to the view that therefore all forms of knowledge will be equally successful in solving a practical problem, equally adequate in explaining a puzzling phenomenon or, in general, equally acceptable to all participants. Nor does it follow that we cannot discriminate between different forms of knowledge with a view to their relevance or adequacy in regard to a specific goal. (Original emphasis)

Another misconception about relativism is that it in some way denies the existence of a real world. This is nonsense. What is argued is that our ways of understanding and describing the world are mediated and partial and that some things are more knowable than others. No one can sensibly argue that reality does not exist. We notice it most when it exerts its malign influence on our lives, it can make us sick and eventually it will kill us. For these reasons a universal constructionist position would be quite untenable. As Hacking (1999: 24) notes in his excellent debunking of the issues, a universal constructionist would be

someone who claims every object whatsoever – the earth, your feet, quarks, the aroma of coffee, grief, polar bears in the Arctic – is in some nontrivial sense socially constructed. Not just our experience of them, our classifications of them, our interests in them, but these things themselves.

Hacking makes an important distinction between different kinds of phenomena that we think can usefully be applied to aspects of clinical judgement. He distinguishes between **indifferent** and **interactive kinds** (of things). Indifferent kinds are natural phenomena like rock, water, oxygen, blood or bones. These phenomena are indifferent to how we describe them. They cannot reinvent themselves as a result. They do not come to see themselves differently as a consequence of how we describe them. Of course, our actions in relation to these indifferent kinds may have unintended consequences – resistant bacteria are a consequence of our use of antibiotics, but the bacteria's resistance is not political! Of course, as we show in Chapter 4, doing science is itself a social business. For example, the interpretation of the results of experiments and so forth may be subject to debate and rely on strategies of argumentation or persuasion, and new ideas may be affected by established ways of thinking. Nevertheless, indifferent kinds are more stable and hence more amenable to being known using scientific method than are interactive kinds.

Interactive kinds include things like our notions of mental illness or child abuse. By describing and understanding mental distress in particular kinds of ways, or defining certain behaviours as abusive, we affect the way those things are experienced by people. They are in that sense 'interactive'. Of course, many things are a combination of indifferent and interactive kinds. The changes in a child's body (for example, bruises, cuts, fractures) following physical assault are indifferent, they simply are. However, in different historical times and cultural spaces they may be defined either as legitimate punishment or as grotesque abuse. In this sense, by calling certain things 'child abuse' we produce an interactive kind. The important thing about interactive kinds is that they have a *moral* dimension. They are often situated on the boundaries of normality and deviance, rightness and wrongness. Moreover, the kinds interact not just with the individuals they describe but with institutions and institutional practices. They are thus of vital importance in understanding professional activity.

Clinical judgement and different kinds

What is the point of all this philosophizing? The point is that clinical judgement, or more particularly case formulation, is a complex business involving both interactive and indifferent phenomena. While EBP and various forms of statistical modelling discussed in Chapter 1 are quite good at interrogating indifferent kinds, and they have considerable transferability to very specific technique-driven psycho-social interventions like cognitive–behavioural therapy, they are sorely deficient at even recognizing the existence of interactive kinds. For example, from where we sit, psychotherapy appears to be almost entirely dependent on interactive kinds. Judgements about what counts as happiness or sadness, adjustment or dysfunction, what makes a relationship healthy, about who is to blame for a person's distress are all emotionally charged and socially mediated. Yet the approach to understanding the practices of therapists has treated the putative 'active ingredients' of therapy as indifferent kinds.

Once we see phenomena as contestable, malleable and relatively subject to change, we need different means through which to interrogate them. In turn, we need to acknowledge that clinicians themselves will need to use different ways of knowing in order to make sense of these phenomena. At these times, emotional and often moral judgements are indispensable. Rather than being a murky contaminant to objectivity, embodied, emoting subjectivity becomes a vital decision-making force. This prospect is only frightening if we cling to the Enlightenment belief that reason and emotion are and should be separate. This view is being increasingly challenged from a number of vantage points. Sociologists like Latour involved in the social study of science have shown that science is itself an alive, contested, sometimes haphazard, emotional, creative business, saturated with social and personal judgements.

However, it is important to avoid oversocializing decision-making. In his work on the discovery of *Helicobactor pylori*, to which we refer in more detail in Chapter 4, Thagard (1999) makes precisely this point. He takes issue with some sociological work on the grounds that it appears to espouse a radically pragmatic view of science, which exaggerates the malleability of reality and truth. He points to the irrefutable causal efficacy of some discoveries. For example, vaccination and antibiotics work because micro-organisms are not simply an invention produced by the germ theory of disease – they really do make people sick. He notes:

> Are scientists deluded in thinking that systematic observation, painstakingly controlled experiments, and rigorous hypothesis evaluation can teach us about the world? The delusion lies instead in those who think that science is just another semiotic exercise like literary criticism or fashion design.
>
> (Thagard 1999: 239)

Thagard's point is well made, but he is constructing a straw man. It is difficult to find an example of the form of radical constructionism he describes.

For example, Bruno Latour comes in for considerable criticism from Thagard, but contrary to popular belief, Latour is not a critic, but an avid fan of his vitalized science (see Chapter 8 and Latour 1999 on the reality of science studies). It is noteworthy that Latour's arguments are very similar to those originating in contemporary neuroscience. For example, the neurologist Antonio Damasio, whose ideas we consider further in Chapter 5, like Latour, wants to recapture an 'embodied mind' and to underscore the essential role that emotion (and the moral judgement associated with it) plays in human reasoning processes. He notes: 'Well-targeted and well-deployed emotion seems to be a support system without which the edifice of reason cannot operate properly' (Damasio 1999: 42). Here, Damasio is arguing, *contra* Descartes, that rationality and emotion are inextricably bound together. Emotions are not the messy and recalcitrant enemies of rationality, but are absolutely integral to the processes of decision-making and judgement. People do not simply think, they intuit, they have 'the feeling of what happens' (Damasio 1999). By placing feelings in their proper role, Damasio and others force us to confront the moral nature of professional practices. This does not, however, mean we can ignore material concerns, dispense with formal knowledge or let feelings run unchecked.

It is with the re-embodied clinician that we are concerned in the chapters that follow. Putting the mind back into a feeling body – that gets angry, has friends, enemies, loyalties, vendettas, has a past and an anticipated future, becomes weary or bored – forces us to consider how we may understand the processes of judgement and intuition more adequately. You remember from

Chapter 1 that the problem with Donald Schön's notion of the intuitive artist was that he did not seem to offer any adequate means by which practitioners could examine their own artistry or 'know how', and decide whether it is good or bad. In the next chapter, we introduce a number of methods for studying and analysing everyday clinical work. We argue that by looking in detail at what clinicians do and by suspending our judgements about whether it is good or bad, we may open for debate some of the aspects of judgement-making that are currently concealed and denied. Our intention is not to provide a critique of clinicians' judgements. That is a job for clinicians and judges. Instead, by pointing to some of the *relativities* in clinical judgement we want to depict it in a more *realistic* way and hence open it up for debate.

Summary

This chapter has argued that:

- Current policy agendas privilege scientific-bureaucratic rationality, best exemplified by EBP.
- In EBP there is a clear hierarchy of evidence, with RCTs as the gold standard.
- EBP oversimplifies or ignores the processes of case formulation, jumping immediately to decisions about treatment and outcome.
- There has been a tendency for RCTs to be applied to activities that do not immediately lend themselves to this type of understanding; for example, social care and psychotherapy.
- In order to understand the robustness of the ideas associated with scientific-bureaucratic rationality we need to examine dominant understandings of truth and knowledge, which originate in the Enlightenment.
- The Enlightenment separation of reason and emotion is only one way of understanding knowledge and truth.
- Certain aspects of clinical work involve complex and morally laden judgements that defy neutral explanation.
- EBP in its current form is eroding appropriate vocabularies by which these judgements may be explored and debated. These need to be developed or resurrected.

3 Interrogating the tacit dimension

Concepts and methods

In the previous two chapters, we argued that clinical judgement involves a good deal of interpretive work. This is the case whether the clinician practises in areas such as pathology or genetics, which may be considered to be more conventionally scientific, or is in the business of making judgements about, and attempting to make a difference to, human emotion or relationships. Once we allow for the possibility of degrees of interpretive flexibility, we also must acknowledge variability in judgement and as a consequence of this variability we must address questions of equity, ethics and morality in more complex ways. For these reasons some authors have reacted against the simplifying tendencies of the scientific-bureaucratic models of professional practice and have called for an understanding of clinical judgement that takes account of 'humaneness' (Little 1995; Downie and Macnaughton 2000). The humane clinician, they argue, requires 'a broad educated perspective' (Downie and Macnaughton 2000: 75) to enable them to make insightful judgements:

> In the clinical situation, I would be insightful if I realised that the patient in front of me really wanted to talk about her concerns about her daughter's drug use rather than the back pain she has officially presented with.
>
> (Downie and Macnaughton 2000: 101)

Through the use of the concept of humaneness, such authors are attempting to reassert the *humanity* of professional activity. In Chapters 1 and 2, we too have asserted that despite attempts to reduce judgement to computer algorithms, case formulation remains a fundamentally human activity, dependent on language, which, in turn, is tied to history and the social world. This leaves us with a problem. We have argued that case formulation relies a good deal on flashes of insight, based on shared understandings, which may be taken for granted and therefore 'tacit'. These forms of judgement are essential and inevitable, but they are not infallible. Moreover, as we noted in Chapter 1, they are likely to be treated as trivial and self-evident and therefore can easily lead to practitioners jumping to conclusions. The tacit dimension has tended to be constructed as in some way unknowable. But it is essential that we consider how it may be opened up for investigation and how clinicians may be assisted to develop a critical perspective upon it. There appear to us to be three main ways in which this problem may be addressed.

- We may look to the humanities for inspiration.
- We may use the insights from various forms of psychoanalysis to interrogate our unconscious motives.
- We may look in detail at what clinicians do and say in the course of their work and attempt to defamiliarize some of the things we take for granted, so that we can discover them anew. By rediscovering what we take for granted, we can decide whether we want to change the ways we think, whether we want to keep them and whether we want to use them on this *particular* occasion in relation to this *particular* case.

We consider these in turn and argue that the third offers a particularly fruitful method for understanding clinical judgement in its social context.

The humanities and humaneness

In the context of medicine, Downie and Macnaughton (2000) and Little (1995) (see also Downie and Charlton 1992) argue for the incorporation into medical training of the study of humanities, particularly literature and philosophy. For example, Downie and Macnaughton (2000: 176) suggest that:

> in demanding an emotional response, the arts allow the reader or viewer to discover their own hidden values and prejudices, and to challenge them. In other words, the arts help students to develop self-awareness and enhance their understanding of the human condition . . . so far in medicine it has been the role of ethics teaching to instruct students on their approach to patients, but an understanding of ethical principles will not develop the sensitivities in the way the study of arts can.

On a similar note, Little (1995: 166) argues that the forms of truth produced by literature have parallels in clinical practice:

> Novelists and poets persuade by over-powering reductionist scientific logic with another dimension of pluralist logic, and we respond with a feeling of truth identified and made manifest. This skill in

> persuasion is part of humanist communication, and it uses a logic different from that of science. There may be no scientific proof of what is said or revealed, but the revelation is no less 'true'. It expresses the truth which resides in ethics, morality and aesthetics.

These ideas are appealing and clearly make sense. For example, Downie and Macnaughton refer to the film *Trainspotting*, arguing that its graphic, tragicomic portrayal of young drug users 'shooting up' does more than any textbook could ever achieve to cast the experiences of 'addiction' in their full human complexity. Similarly, studying history may well help to give context to current ways of understanding normality and deviance or pathology, and illustrate the way in which thinking shifts over time. We agree that incorporating the humanities into professional education and development can do only good. However, while the arts offer a means to examine emotion and thus can provide some kind of pathway both to self-knowledge and to understanding the human condition, they do not offer a means for practitioners systematically to interrogate their own practice. We are still left with the problem of how to develop a rigorous approach to Schön's reflection-on-action.

Psychoanalysis and self-knowledge

As a means to develop this rigour, it seems tempting to turn to psychoanalysis, which claims quite explicitly to develop critical self-awareness. It sets out to examine the emotional aspects of human existence and challenges the idea of uncontaminated rationality (see Frosh 1997 for a helpful review of debates in psychoanalysis). The concepts associated with the reflective practice movement (see Chapter 1) rely implicitly on the idea of a dynamic unconscious, which may be influencing our judgements about particular cases. The problem with psychoanalysis is that it is a discipline with its own range of concepts and explanatory frameworks, which are very powerful and seductive. Psychoanalysis superimposes its own order on human activity by using powerful metaphors which, when used therapeutically may be very potent, but in the context of research may conceal more than they reveal.

That is, psychoanalysis starts from a very clearly defined theoretical position, which is virtually incorrigible because 'psychoanalysts can wriggle out of anything by appealing to the trickery of the unconscious' (Frosh 1997: 234). So psychoanalytic accounts, while accepting and indeed celebrating the essential emotionality and subjectivity of human reason, always and necessarily claim privilege for their own version – they know best because they have access to the superior knowledge of *your* subconscious provided for them by the theory. For example, in a text on research methods, Hollway and Jefferson (2000) argue that psychoanalytic ideas associated with the work of Melanie Klein (for a summary see Grosskurth 1986) may usefully be incorporated into certain forms of qualitative research, particularly those that explore individual accounts of human experiences, such as oral history and life story work. Klein's ideas are very complex, but basically incorporate a view of the 'self' as a product of unconscious defences against anxiety, which begin in early infancy. The outcome of these struggles may result in one of two principal perspectives on the world: the paranoid-schizoid, which construes the world in terms of contrasts between good and bad, and the depressive, which allows us to see things as a mixture of good and bad.

In their empirical work, Hollway and Jefferson investigate fear of crime in a neighbourhood. As a result of their theoretical starting point, they impose particular categories on the accounts given by their subjects, classifying and interpreting their stories as examples of either depressive or paranoid-schizoid positions. That is, Hollway and Jefferson tell *Kleinian* stories about the stories their subjects have told. For example, one of their subjects, 'Roger', tells them a story about his experiences of crime on the estate, which Hollway and Jefferson classify as evidence of an unconscious paranoid-schizoid position in which Roger is 'splitting off' the bad parts of himself. They warrant this by referring to two aspects of Roger's story, first his idealization of the past and second his assertion that he is frightened of walking around the estate after dark. He accounts for this fear by recounting stories of various muggings, for which he says 'Jamaicans' were to blame. He refers also to Scots and gypsies on the estate. Roger's 'them and us' version is rewritten by Hollway and Jefferson as an example of 'paranoid-schizoid' splitting. This ignores the social dimension of storytelling and the fact that narratives of personal troubles are moral affairs that must be seen in relation to historical and cultural time (Reissman 2001).

Hollway and Jefferson use a Kleinian-shaped template to carve out a meaning in their subjects' stories. This gives the stories a form and content that they did not originally possess. We doubt that Hollway and Jefferson shared their theoretical interest with their informants. If they had, they may have elicited different accounts. So what was Roger trying to accomplish with his particular telling of the troubles? Rather than imputing deep psychological structures, if we stay with the features of the story itself, we might want to see Roger's account as a display of his own positive moral identity, accomplished by drawing on cultural ideas common on the estate. The only warrant for Hollway and Jefferson's reinterpretation of Roger's story is psychoanalytic thought itself. While denying any claims to have captured absolute truth, the authors repeatedly assert the correctness of their interpretations, again using the theory as evidence. The problem is that their interpretations cannot be empirically validated. They are convincing only to those readers who share a belief in the intrinsic correctness of their particular theory. It is an entirely circular analysis. The effect of this rewriting is to underexplore the narratives that their subjects produce. This is a common problem with psychological theory and is a point we take up in more detail in Chapter 4.

Obviously psychoanalysis has its uses. Indeed, we hope that some of the readers of this book will be psychotherapists of various kinds. However, rather than using psychoanalysis as a means to examine judgements, we would argue that the metaphors and stories it produces demand interrogation in their own right. If we want to be more realistic about clinical practice and to explore how it gets done, we will need to avoid rewriting people's activities, accounts and expressed opinions and motivations. Instead we will need to look in more detail at what clinicians do in their day-to-day activities, at their ways of talking and writing about their cases and at the effects of these activities. There is a pressing need for clinicians and educators to interrogate the processes of persuasion and argument involved in case formulation in more detail, as these are at the heart of understanding what is taken for granted in practice.

Interpretive social science and the sociology of everyday life

In this book, we want to encourage you to become intrigued by what is known already – that is, by those thoughts and actions that have become so familiar and taken for granted in your everyday practice that you are no longer aware of them. Being astounded and fascinated by the everyday should not remain an exclusive pleasure of social scientists! We argue that by looking at professional talk and work in context we can see how the tacit dimensions, the qualitative aspects of judgement, can be made visible, available and reportable and how they sit alongside and invoke 'knowledge' in its traditionally understood, objective and stable sense.

There are a number of concepts and methods associated with a branch of human science often referred to as interpretivism, which social scientists have used to interrogate the cultures and practices of health professionals in precisely the way we describe above. However, as we noted in Chapter 2, there is evidence that the 'gold-standard' methodologies, associated with the scientific-bureaucratic model and the narrowly defined current version of EBP, are squeezing out these approaches and hence are leaving areas of clinical practice immune from analysis and understanding, as Webb (2001: 62–3) notes:

> The kinds of research methodology which are considered favourable in providing evidence are random control trials, single case experimentation, double-blind and cohort studies, and crossover designs. Checklists of evidence indicators are recommended to practitioners

to ensure the reliability and validity of the research. It is interesting, but hardly surprising that no mention is made of other main-stream research methods which are taught on sociology and cultural studies course, such as ethnography, discourse analysis, actor network theory, semiotics or psychoanalysis. Presumably these more interpretive methodologies which continue to make a significant impact on contemporary social sciences are considered either too subjective, lacking in cost-effectiveness or the disciplinary prestige of the medical sciences.

We now introduce some of the methods Webb describes and argue for their practical utility in the context of professional education and practice. As Webb's list illustrates, interpretivism is a broad church incorporating a range of disciplinary, philosophical and methodological positions. We cannot hope to do justice to the whole range here, and our more modest purpose is to introduce you to some relevant ideas to enable you to make more sense of subsequent chapters. However, some suggestions for further reading are given at the end of the book. Before we outline some of the specific orientations and methodologies associated with interpretivism we must consider what kinds of phenomena it is attempting to understand.

The methods associated with interpretivism tend to elicit descriptive accounts of how a particular cultural group, such as Trobriand Islanders in the Pacific (Malinowski 1922), disaffected youth (Whyte 1981), doctors (for example, Strong 1979; Silverman 1987; Atkinson 1995), nurses (Latimer 2000) or social workers (for example, Hall 1997; White 1999, 2001), go about constructing and making sense of their lives. The primary concern of research conducted in this tradition is to describe in detail the everyday, routine practices of certain groups. The anthropologist Clifford Geertz (1973) has used the expression 'thick description' to describe this way of representing reality.

An aim in most interpretive work is that the reasoning of the researcher should be 'inductive'; that is, derived from the data and the understandings of the 'members' (subjects of the study) rather than from a particular hypothesis or theory. However, no research can ever be entirely without presupposition, and it is perfectly possible that a qualitative researcher may, in a sense, be testing theory. Qualitative research has now generated a substantial cumulative knowledge base, and by setting out to see whether the practices described by a researcher at one time in one setting are also evident in other times and places, researchers may very clearly be testing theory (*inter alia* Hammersley 1992; Silverman 1997, 2000). Nevertheless, the *aspiration* to inductivism, to *generating* hypotheses *from* data, differs substantively from the hypothetico-deductive reasoning of pharmacological and other biomedical research, and from psychoanalytic thinking, which is primarily theoretically driven. Interpretive research, then, is concerned with answering 'What's going on here?' or 'How does this or that get done?' sorts of questions. The research questions tend not to speculate in great detail about what might be found. They do not necessarily consist of falsifiable hypotheses, but instead seek to explore and provide a representation of 'what's going on' in the clinics, wards, corridors and meeting rooms of this particular setting.

In keeping with the preference for inductive reasoning, interpretive studies often eschew taking a 'normative' position in relation to the people or activity they are investigating. That is, they are not oriented to exposing error, taking up a cause or fighting the corner of any underdog, although clearly when others read their studies these may be potential outcomes. Their orientation is not to evaluation but to description. There are exceptions to this, such as some forms of action, emancipatory or feminist research (*inter alia* Stanley 1990; Truman *et al.* 2000), which may be oriented to particular political ends, such as exposing or changing discriminatory aspects of women's health care. Illuminating though such work can be, the studies we have drawn upon in this book generally do not adopt any such normative view, but instead set out to represent what clinicians do in their day-to-day work. For example, we have omitted entirely any studies that presuppose the relevance of, and reduce everything to, a simplistically formulated theory of 'oppression'. Our reasons are expressed pithily by Silverman (2000: 70):

> Just as doctors talk about meeting patients who make their hearts sink, there is nothing worse than when a detailed seminar on one's research is greeted by some bright spark with a version of: 'That's all very interesting. But surely what you've described is all to do with power/gender/postmodernity etc.' What a nice simple world it would be if everything could be reduced to one factor! For the moment, however, we should leave the pursuit of this kind of simplicity to bigots.

Normative and prescriptive judgements on practice have their place. Patients, managers or auditors, for example, may very properly make them. However, it is our view that research should be encouraged, which is sufficiently detailed to allow these judgements to be made by the clinicians themselves. This kind of self-evaluation is unlikely to be encouraged by an incursion of solemn social researchers with little interest in clinicians' daily grind, who are hell-bent on exposing errant or 'oppressive' practices.

Table 3.1 summarizes (and obviously simplifies) some of the differences between interpretivism and what, for the sake of comparison, we have called the positivist paradigm, which could include any methodology concerned with uncovering linear relations of causation.

You will remember that in Chapter 2 we discussed Hacking's (1999) distinction between 'interactive' and 'indifferent' kinds. It should now be clear

Table 3.1 Differences between the interpretive and positivist paradigms

Interpretive paradigm	Positivist paradigm
Usually advocates qualitative methods	Usually advocates quantitative methods
Concerned with understanding phenomena from the actor's perspective	Seeks to uncover relations of causation
Naturalistic – prefers 'naturally occurring', uncontrolled settings	Controlled measurement
A degree of subjectivity or interpretation is acknowledged as inevitable	objective
Close to data – insider	Removed from data – outsider
Inductive, grounded, exploratory, descriptive – concerned with meanings	Hypothetico-deductive, confirmatory, predictive
Process-oriented	Outcome-oriented
Valid, real, rich and deep	Reliable, hard, replicable
Generates theory that may be transferable to and should be explicit enough to be testable in other settings	Aims to be generalizable
Assumes a contingent, dynamic, layered reality	Assumes that the reality (or the thing) it is investigating can be made fixed and stable, like the dosage of a drug

Source: adapted from Reichardt and Cook (1979).

that the left-hand side of Table 3.1 is likely to provide methods more suited to exploring 'interactive' kinds, which are laden with situated social meanings. We have argued that research in health and social care, and hence our understandings of clinical judgement, are becoming increasingly monopolized by the right-hand side of Table 3.1, which is well placed to investigate 'indifferent' kinds like human anatomy and physiology and the actions of drugs upon them. Of course, many areas of clinical practice have a reasonable 'fit' with this kind of inquiry. However, for many others this is not the case. Indeed, many aspects of health care appear to be straightforwardly concerned with 'indifferent' kinds, but are actually much more contestable, once we look at them in new ways. Let us consider a dramatic example – death – surely an irrefutable, indifferent fact of life.

Death is one of the classic examples given by scholars who want to argue against the ideas associated with social constructionism (see Edwards *et al.* 1995 and Potter *et al.* 1999 for a more detailed debunking of such 'death and furniture' arguments). 'People die,' the argument goes. 'That can't be socially constructed. When I'm dead I'm dead, if you're such a clever social constructionist, resurrect me!' Of course, death is a simple truth, a biological fact, but looked at through an interpretive lens, we can see that there are degrees of flexibility about whether and when someone is so classified, as Silverman (2000: 81) notes:

> in 1963, after President Kennedy was shot, he was taken to Dallas hospital with, according to contemporary accounts, half his head shot away. My hunch is that if you or I were to arrive in this state, we would be given a cursory examination and then recorded as 'dead on arrival' (DOA). Precisely because they were dealing with a President, the staff had to do more than this. So they worked on Kennedy for almost an hour, demonstrating thereby that they had done their best for such an important patient.

None of these procedures, of course, could revive the President, whose death remained a material reality, but it demonstrates that the decision about whether someone is certified 'DOA' may be something one could investigate in its own right. In this way, Sudnow (1968) and Glaser and Strauss (1965, 1968) devoted their studies to the social organization of dying, without, of course, being forced thereby to deny that dying happens.

Rather than seeking to refute the reality of death, such studies reveal its ritual and often deeply moral aspects. For example, in her more recent work on representations of death, Bradbury (1999: 53) notes the moral importance of age. She cites the following extract:

> [We feel worse] if they are young, like someone [who dies] giving birth by Caesarean, or someone who has died a couple of days after a massive car crash. Because in fact, life is much more sacred, I suppose when they are younger. Obviously. Much cheaper when you are old. (Charlotte, doctor)

Similarly, Bloor's (1994) study of variations in death certification practices showed how doctors attended to moral imperatives, such as sparing the relatives' grief, in certifying the cause of death.

It is rather the same with something like child abuse. We can, and obviously should, treat abuse as a material fact. Clearly children are abused, sometimes brutally, horribly, fatally. However, when a case is referred to a social services department, the decision about whether it should be treated as a child protection investigation, rather like the DOA example, is a good deal more complicated than it may first appear. Of course, the decision has no effect on what has already happened to the child – that simply 'is' – but it has a great deal of effect on how that event is classified and on what is done about it. Like those associated with death, these kinds of decision carry massive moral weight and often depend on evaluations of the moral status of the parties in the case (see Chapter 5). We can therefore investigate them using the methods of interpretivism, *as well as* looking for clinical indicators of child abuse.

We began this section by noting that interpretive social science is a broad church. We have already made some points about the sorts of research we use in the chapters that follow, but in order for you to make sense of these we need to say a little more about the kinds of methods the studies have used. So what specific kinds of research may be most useful to us in opening up the more qualitative and 'tacit' dimensions of clinical judgement?

Deep familiarity: the ethnographic case study

> In its most characteristic form [ethnography] involves the ethno-grapher participating, overtly or covertly, in people's daily lives for an extended period of time, watching what happens, listening to what is said, asking questions – in fact, collecting whatever data are available to throw light on the issues that are the focus of the research.
>
> (Hammersley and Atkinson 1995: 1–2)

Here, in what has become a classic text on the ethnographic method, Hammersley and Atkinson mark out the basic features of ethnographic inquiry. With its roots in anthropology, ethnography has much in common with the methods we use routinely to make sense of our world as social beings. When, as professionals, we embark upon training and are sent out on practice or clinical placements it is as amateur ethnographers that we confront the confusing organizational context of the occupation we have chosen. We have to try to work out what it is we are supposed to be doing; who is considered to be competent in the organization and why; whom we should avoid; where the notes are stored; when and how to write in them, what the abbreviations mean and so forth. It is with these everyday contingencies that ethnography is concerned, as Goffman (1961: ix–x) notes:

> any group of persons – prisoners, primitives, pilots, or patients – develop a life of their own that becomes meaningful, reasonable and normal once you get close to it, and . . . a good way to learn about any of these worlds is to submit oneself in the company of the members to the daily round of petty contingencies to which they are subject.

So when they produce their 'thick descriptions' ethnographers are trying to render explicit to members of one cultural setting what it is like to be part of another. Ethnographic accounts, however, have the potential to make members of the original setting see their own work in a new light. This has particular implications for our project in this book. If ethnographic research is focused on the everyday, then it may help clinicians to make sense of what Schön calls 'knowing-in-action' (see Chapter 1), as Bloor (1997: 223) notes:

> [Social] research which takes practitioners' everyday work as its topical focus: social research which seeks to describe and compare practitioners' everyday work practices self-evidently invites practitioners to juxtapose and weigh their own practices with those reported by the researcher.

In short, analytic ethnography may help to defamiliarize (Aull Davies 1999; White 2001) some taken-for-granted aspects of practice and hence make these amenable to debate and analysis.

Ethnography carries with it all sorts of claims to authenticity, deep familiarity and 'intimate knowledge' (Mitchell 1983: 207) with one or a limited number of settings, which, it is argued, allow researchers to make theoretical claims that may be transferable with care to other settings. Brewer (1994: 236) defines his commitment to ethnography thus,

> The belief that fragments of recorded talk, extracts from fieldnotes, and reports of observed actions can reliably represent a social world . . . [and] that small scale, micro events in everyday life have at least common features with the broader social world, such that general processes permeate down to and are in part reproduced at the level of people's everyday lives. Thus microscopic events can illustrate features of broader social processes, so long as the ethnographer sets out the grounds on which these empirical generalizations are made.

Here we can see hints to some of the debates internal to ethnography that are beyond the scope of this book, but that concern the transparency and theoretical lucidity of the ethnographer's analyses (for further detail see, *inter alia*, Atkinson 1990; Hammersley 1992; Brewer 1994). This is not the place for a detailed critical appraisal of ethnography as a research method, but suffice it to say that there has been increasing attention paid to the ways in which ethnographers establish the validity and reliability of their findings. The purpose of ethnography is to explicate the shared cultural aspects of a particular setting. Thus, ethnographic accounts depend substantially on the ethnographer's techniques of data presentation and persuasion.

As readers, we do not have access to the site of the ethnography (although clearly health or welfare professionals may have knowledge of similar settings), so how do we know that they are true? In recent decades substantial work has taken place that sets out criteria by which ethnographic work may be evaluated. Many of these concern the meanings that the ethnographer places on people's talk and actions in the setting.

This concern has led to a variety of ethnographic subspecies, and one subclassification provided by Silverman (1993) is particularly useful for understanding the nature of the studies we have drawn upon in this book. Silverman distinguishes between what he calls **interactionist** and **ethnomethodological** ethnographic traditions. The first is concerned with the *meanings* actors in a setting ascribe to their practices. The problem with this is that meanings are not immediately observable, because they are essentially psychological states and the actions themselves may be ambiguous. It may thus lead the ethnographer into the kinds of rewriting we saw in Hollway and Jefferson's psychoanalytic work, which we considered earlier in this chapter. Thus, just as the clinician has a high degree of interpretive flexibility in deciding what is wrong with a patient who presents with ambiguous symptoms, the ethnographer may also interpret actions to mean a range of different things.

Ethnographers within the interactionist tradition argue that deep familiarity with the setting, along with a set of techniques for testing interpretations, such as seeking the views of members of the setting, looking for disconfirming evidence and so forth, helps to ensure that correct interpretations are made. Nevertheless, these criticisms have led to a shift in focus away from cultural meanings and on to what is *observable* in the setting and particularly on to the talk taking place and the documents and written accounts produced. This type of study is generally known as ethnomethodological ethnography. We have drawn on both types of study in this book, but it is worth looking at the influence of ethnomethodology in more detail, as we think this holds considerable potential for helping clinicians to add rigour to their attempts to undertake 'reflection-on-action'.

Ordinary action: ethnomethodology and conversation analysis

The term **ethnomethodology** was first used by Harold Garfinkel (1967), and simply means 'folk (ethno) methods (ways of doing things)'. Ethnomethodology provides a means to analyse and explore the ways in which people make sense of and reproduce ordinary, everyday social practices. It seeks to move away from judging whether a particular practice is right or wrong, to look instead at how that practice gets done and what practical action(s) makes it work. This approach has had a very significant impact on ethnography as Maynard notes:

> [Ethnographers] have traditionally asked – 'How do participants see things?' – [with] the presumption that reality lies outside the words spoken in a particular time and place. The [alternative] question – 'How do participants do things?' – suggests that the micro social order can be appreciated more fully by studying how speech and other face-to-face behaviours *constitute* reality within actual mundane situations.
>
> (Maynard 1989: 144, emphasis added)

This emphasis on observable action actually *constituting* the setting is crucial. We need to look not beneath or behind the action, but at how the action itself produces order, culture and other taken-for-granted aspects of the setting. Along with the timely invention of reliable recording equipment, this focus on the routine and mundane has led to the use of transcripts of talk in ethnographic work, of which we have made considerable use in chapters that follow (see also Taylor and White 2000).

The emphasis on language or 'talk' in ethnomethodology is important and is a consequence of the special importance placed on the **accounts** people produce of and for their actions. Accounts *of* events also usually embody some kind justification *for* the action taken. So, in ethnomethodology, what people say cannot be taken as an unproblematic reflection of what really happened. Social actors thus make complex decisions about what they say or do on the basis of certain norms of behaviour and, thus, the accounts given in any situation will draw on tacit knowledge about the moral order in which the encounter is located. The way in which the account is constructed will be determined by the context in which the talk takes place. In the selection of account, therefore, social actors will draw on shared understandings about how a competent individual (sociologist, friend, nurse, social worker, therapist, doctor, health visitor) should properly behave under a given set of circumstances.

This insight has led interview data to be treated in different ways: not as a means to access authentic experience about being a mother, a gay man, an older person placed in a nursing home or a patient on a urology ward, but as a socially situated account that is constructed in a particular way and draws on shared understandings about how one should properly 'be' any of these things. It may be helpful to consider an example of this way of reading interviews as 'texts'. Dorothy Smith's (1978) seminal sociological paper on the ways in which people use language to signal deviance in another is a useful illustration. In the interview analysed by Smith, a student is describing to an interviewer (a fellow student), the behaviour of one of her friends, 'K'. Smith's analysis is lengthy and detailed and the transcript of the interview runs to several pages. This extract is, therefore, simply a 'taster'.

> My recognition that there might be something wrong was very gradual, and I was actually the last of her close friends who was openly willing to admit that she was becoming mentally ill ... We would go to the beach or the pool on a hot day, and I would sort of dip in and just lie in the sun, while K insisted that she had to swim 30 lengths.
>
> (Smith 1978: 28)

We are being invited by the student (Angela), and indeed by the interviewer who supports Angela's version, to believe that K is mentally ill. Like the ethnomethodologists, we want you to suspend judgement for the moment on whether or not this is so and to concentrate instead on the organization of Angela's account. First, note that certain expectations are set up. It is suggested that K was becoming mentally ill, but that Angela was the last of her close friends to accept this. This has the effect of casting Angela as a witness to events who is reluctant to see what is clear to others – that K is mentally ill. In making this statement Angela reinforces the plausibility of her version, signalling that she had to be confronted with overwhelming evidence before making her judgement. As she has the privileged status as witness to the events, she would be difficult to challenge unless the challenger had also been present on the occasions she reports.

In Smith's terms, these techniques help to 'authorize' Angela's version. This gives Angela **definitional privilege** – the power to define. It is her behaviour and not K's that provides the norm (for example, 'We would go to the beach or the pool on a hot day, and I would sort of dip in and just lie in the sun, while K insisted that she had to swim 30 lengths'). As Smith points out, none of the behaviours described by Angela, intrinsically provide evidence that K is mentally ill. Smith notes that some descriptions of K's behaviour may indeed be read as strengths (swimming 30 lengths) were it not for the skilful work of the teller of the tale. By the careful assembly of the facts of K's behaviour, as readers or hearers, we are led to see her responses 'as arising from a state of the individual and not as motivated by her by features of her situation' (Smith 1978: 38). Contextual information is assembled so that K's behaviour does not appear understandable in the circumstances or motivated by her rational analysis of the situation.

Smith calls these strategies **contrast structures**. In a contrast structure, the first part of the statement sets up an expectation, in this instance provided by Angela, who has the power to define, while the other(s) signal(s) deviation from this expectation. For example:

1   'We would go down to the beach on a hot day' (this identifies the context of the action and hence allows the reader to make predictions about what sort of behaviour is appropriate).

2 'I would sort of dip in and just lie in the sun' (this provides an example of normal behaviour as prescribed by the person with *definitional privilege*).

3 'While K insisted that she had to swim 30 lengths' (here, K's behaviour, which may otherwise be considered appropriate activity for a beach, is contrasted with the norm set by Angela and is also presented as obsessional by the use of the words 'insisted that she had to').

In later chapters, we make use of Smith's work contrast structures and show that they are ubiquitous in professional accounts, where they are often used to shore up the more contestable aspects of clinical judgement.

The interest in talk spawned by ethnomethodology led to the creation of a new discipline: **conversation analysis** (CA). This is associated particularly with the work of Harvey Sacks (e.g. 1972, 1992; or, for a more accessible summary, Silverman 1998). The recognition that language was about more than description and that it actually performed things led to a search for empirical methods that could record and analyse instances of talk. The attention in CA is on the sequential features of talk; that is, the turns people take, the pauses in the talk, the way new topics are introduced and so forth (see Sacks *et al.* 1974). CA uses very detailed transcripts (an example of transcription symbols is given in the Appendix), which attempt to represent as much of the 'real time' talk as possible. Often unconventional spellings are used to indicate regional accent and pauses are recorded in tenths of a second, along with laughs, coughs, outbreaths and what are known as 'non-lexical vocalizations' (such as erm, or ahh) (see West 1996 for a discussion of transcripts and transcription in research). These methods have facilitated the detailed analysis of particular types of encounter, such as those taking place between doctors and patients. The rich detail of the transcripts produced in CA can be very revealing, as Silverman notes in relation to a study by Clavarino *et al.* (1995), concerned with establishing whether cancer patients had understood prognostic statements telling them that their condition was fatal:

> When researchers first listened to the tapes . . . they sometimes felt there was no evidence that the patients had picked up their doctors' often guarded statements about their prognosis. However, when the tapes were retranscribed [using conversation analytic symbols] it was demonstrated that patients often used very soft utterances (like 'yes' or more usually 'mm') to mark that they were taking up this information. Equally, doctors would monitor patients' silences and rephrase their prognosis statements.
>
> (Silverman 2000: 10)

CA has also been important in showing the moral dimensions of people's talk. For example, in an analysis of interviewees' accounts of their marital breakdown and of radio discussions of family troubles involving family members and counsellors, Cuff (1993) shows that it is common for family members to produce different and competing versions of events and often to blame each other. He shows that the tellers of these versions are oriented to the moral dimensions of their own and others' stories, such that members would not stick rigidly to their version come what may. On the contrary, they produced a variety of contingent versions that did particular moral work and linked sequentially back to other members' statements made earlier in the discussion. Thus, Cuff reveals that family members' versions of their troubles not only do moral work for the teller but are also contingent, incomplete, interdependent and unfolding gradually over a number of turns. That is, they are not pre-made versions of truth, but are actively and collaboratively produced in the setting. The counsellors, for the immediate practical purposes of advice giving, could be seen constructing their own 'expert' versions of the troubles, selectively incorporating elements from individual members' versions. We show similar processes in our extended case study in Chapter 7.

Membership categorization: talking morality

For understanding the moral dimensions of people's talk, Sacks's conversation analytic work on what he calls **membership categorization** analysis is particularly important (*inter alia* Sacks 1972, 1992; Silverman 1998). Sacks argues that, along with other sequential features of talk, the use of social categories such as 'mother' or 'child' can operate as a means of referencing deviance or normality (Jayussi 1991; Housley and Fitzgerald 2002). Often a number of social categories may plausibly be applied to an individual. We often see this in newspaper reports. Silverman gives the following example:

> As feminists have pointed out women, but not men, tend to be identified by their marital status, number of children, hair colour and even chest measurement. Such identifications, while intelligible, carry massive implications for the sense we attach to people and their behaviour. Compare, for example, 'Shapely blonde mother of five' with 'Thirty-two year old teacher'. Both descriptions may 'accurately' describe different aspects of the same person, but each constitutes very definitely how we are to view that person.
>
> (Silverman 1998: 79)

Membership categories are associated with certain activities (**category bound activities**, CBAs), and by describing behaviour that either conforms or fails to conform with these expectations we may establish positive or negative moral identities. So, if 'mother' is associated with nurturance and care, a description of behaviours departing from these expectations will serve to reference deviance. Membership categories are in turn associated with **membership categorization devices** (MCDs), so the categories 'mother' and 'child' are part of the membership categorization device 'family', whereas 'teacher' is a category of the device 'occupation'. Some categories tend to occur in pairs, signalling mutual rights, duties or obligations (mother love, children need), of which mother–child and doctor–patient are examples. These pairings are termed **standardized relational pairs** (SRPs). Often membership categories are explicitly stated (for example, this is a patient), but sometimes they are referenced by association to some activity or attribute associated with a category (for example, I have observed these symptoms). That is, categorization can be done by invoking the *predicates* of a category, as Housley (2000: 104–5) notes:

> if the topic was the moral evaluation of an individual, one might state 'I don't like him/her, s/he is a bad person' . . . or one might refer to the same person as being 'lazy', recount stories of their behaviour on previous occasions (they drank too much at a party), or suggest that their outward appearance conceals some dark motives (for example, their eyes are too close together, etc.). In both cases these strategies can be used to do various types of work within *occasioned* settings.

Professionals routinely use both categories and predicates of categories in their judgements, and these categorizations do important work within clinical settings. The following example is taken from White's (2002) study of paediatrics. The setting is a briefing session between a consultant paediatrician and a registrar prior to an outpatient clinic:

Extract 3.1

Cons: Matthew Long

Reg: [Mmm]

Cons: He's been in with asthma but that's not why he comes to see us (.4). The main reason is some hydronephrosis – I think I've got the last (), seems to have a problem attending [reading]. Repeat ultrasound October 99, it's still hydronephrosis, further up (.5) urinary tract infection, yeah, for definite.

Reg: That's back in (.) April

Cons: Back in April. DMSA [dimercaptosuccinic acid – test to assess scarring and relative function of kidney] clear. Mild right sided hydronephrosis with prominent renal pelvis mainly extra renal, no

scarring and (.) no (.) reflux. (.7) So, I suppose I thought that the best way was to do repeat the ultrasound if the kidney was blowing up and we needed a (), so that's fine. It's difficult sometimes with these mild hydronephrosis. You never know whether it's the beginning of –
Reg: Or whether it's borderline –
Cons: Or whether it's just the [way] they're made –
Reg: [Yeah] yeah

We can see that the patient is identified first by his name, 'Matthew Long', but thereafter the account is 'depersonalized' (Anspach 1988) with reference to the diagnostic categories asthma and hydronephrosis. References to charac-ter(istics) in this account are confined to the interior of Matthew's body. Although Matthew could have been categorized as a child, here he remains in the membership category 'patient', which means that his pathology is relevant but, for example, other categories in the device 'family' are not. However, the following example taken from the same briefing session is very different:

Extract 3.2
Cons: Right let's just see what this was. (2.0) This is a child (.) who – (.) came to see Dr Ross urgency of micturition [passing urine], very, very nervous (.) erm father was the carer. Parents were split up mother with new partner, two younger sisters. No warning when wees (3.0) I think was like an underlying message that parents were split up and father was the carer and I think she was just a bit worried that there were alternative psycho-social agendas, which were not explicit
Reg: Rrrright

Here the paediatrician begins by referring to the category child and moves quickly into providing biographical and family details. In the context of paediatrics this signals that the zone of relevance for clinical activity may lie beyond the child's body in her family relationships. The phrase 'father was the carer' is used twice, the second time immediately before referrence to possible 'alternative psycho-social agendas'. This is heard as meaningful by the registrar and both clinicians draw on their shared domain-specific knowledge that problems with wetting can be associated with trauma, includ-ing sexual abuse. Thus, the categories used in paediatrics constitute cases as either medical or social, signalling the zone of relevance for further inquiry (White 2002). They can also be powerful devices for accomplishing **blamings**.

So we can see that CA studies clearly have importance for understanding how clinical judgements are made and communicated. However, paradoxic-ally, the rich turn-by-turn detail that CA can provide can also be its limitation. It is very difficult to analyse long extracts of talk in this way and a good deal of professional talk takes place in the form of monologues, consisting of long narrative passages; for example, where a patient is giving or a clinician is reporting a history. To study this kind of talk, researchers may make use of a range of techniques associated with an interdisciplinary field known as discourse studies.

Storytelling in clinical practice: discourse studies

Discourse studies comprises a number of disciplines and research traditions, each with its own vast literature. For our present purposes we want to introduce you to the conceptual resources of those traditions that might inform the investigation of professional work. These include ethnomethodology and conversation analysis, which we have discussed above, but also **discursive psychology** and **Foucauldian discourse analysis**.

The strength of CA is that it describes how people work up social reality in the turn-by-turn pattern of conversation. However, the limitation of CA for understanding clinical work is that it risks neglecting the functions of longer sequences of talk and the wider socio-cultural context in which storytelling occurs. To understand the functions and effects of storytelling in clinical work we have to take account of both the proximal (turn-by-turn) and distal (social, cultural and historical) influences on the talk in the clinical setting. The hybrid discipline of discursive psychology, arising from a critique of the traditional cognitive paradigm in social psychology, appears to have something to offer in this respect.

Inspired by ethnomethodology, and borrowing from CA and interactional sociolinguistics (for example, Brown and Levinson 1987), discursive psychology has several prominent exponents (Billig 1991; Edwards and Potter 1992; Marks 1993; Shotter 1993). Although grounded in talk-in-interaction, it also views knowledge and reality as contested and potentially political projects. In this sense it shares some features of a form of discourse analysis associated with Michel Foucault (see, for example, 1973, 1976, 1980). Foucault also views language as something that does more than describe objects and events. He, too, sees it as something that structures, constructs or produces 'reality'. However, Foucault is concerned with the ways in which certain ideas (what he calls 'regimes of truth') have the capacity to make us think, feel and do particular things. After Foucault, discursive psychology is interested in the ways in which people use cultural systems of theoretical, moral and practical beliefs, norms and ideologies; that is, in how they use resources beyond the local interactive details of talk itself, to warrant their reality and knowledge claims. Thus, it takes into account texts and discourses of society at large, but also looks at how these are strategically mobilized to authorize particular versions of social reality.

For example, when a clinician makes use of the diagnostic category Munchausen syndrome by proxy (for example, Meadow 1980, 1985), which is the production by a parent or carer of factitious illness in a child, or exaggeration or exacerbation of an existing condition (see Chapter 6), they draw upon cultural resources, which originate outside the encounter with the patient. These are tied in turn to moral ideas about proper parenthood, such as what constitutes a normal, acceptable degree of anxiety about the health of one's child and what constitutes pathological 'illness behaviour'. These factors are not invented within the conversation the doctor is having with the patient, or with his or her colleagues about the case. Obviously they will be reproduced in the talk and the clinician must manage the turn-by-turn contingencies of the encounter. Yet if we are to understand the detailed judgements clinicians make about their cases in their full complexity, we must consider why certain formulations may 'work' now, while they may have been considered preposterous in the past. So, the naming of a specific syndrome 'Munchausen syndrome by proxy' makes a formulation such as 'I think this woman has put her own blood in the child's urine in order to provoke a professional response' seem worthy of further investigation, when 30 years ago it may have seemed extremely far-fetched.

To give a further example, Carl May (1992a, b) uses Foucault's ideas to show how concepts about the psychological impact of terminal illness, alongside notions of holistic nursing, have extended the domain of nursing practice into psychosocial aspects of patient care. He notes:

> nurses are now required to extend their 'gaze' beyond the concrete condition of the body, and to intrude into patients' private, subjective sphere . . . The patient's uncertainties, anxieties and suspicions about, for example, her possible prognosis are now explicitly defined in terms of *psychosocial problems* which form a new sphere in nursing work . . . In the case of terminal illness, the anxieties and distress that are experienced by patients have taken on a formal symptomatology and have been reconstituted as problems to be resolved.
>
> (May 1992a: 591–2, original emphasis)

This extension, while apparently progressive, may expose patients to evaluative judgements about, for example, whether they are adjusting properly to their illness. So the historical focus of Foucault's work can help us to think about why some ideas are powerful and some are not, and how this potency shifts over time.

Thus, the eclectic field of discourse analysis offers concepts and resources with which to approach the analysis of storytelling in professional practice. For example, Stancombe (2002), using a combination of turn-by-turn analysis and more Foucauldian ideas, has shown how family therapists tend to try to shift accountability for family troubles away from children or young people and towards parents. We show this in more detail in Chapters 5 and 7. This is observable in the transcripts of the talk, but it cannot be fully understood without looking at cultural constructions of childhood as a time of passivity and vulnerablility (Rose 1989, 1998; Stainton Rogers and Stainton Rogers 1992; Burman 1994). These constructions have been particularly dominant in child health and welfare work for some decades and are now reflected in the law and in professional discourses (Dingwall and Murray 1983; Marks 1995; White 1998, 2001, 2002).

By providing analytic devices with real practical utility, discourse analysis can help to move professional practice beyond both technique-driven mechanistic practice and benign introspective reflection. In the chapters that follow we use our own and others' ethnographic and discourse analytic studies to show how they can help us to be more realistic about clinical judgement in context.

Summary

In this chapter we have argued that:

- Research based on experimental methodologies can only take us so far in understanding clinical judgement. To interrogate its more qualitative aspects we need insights generated by the human sciences.
- While the humanities can help a great deal in providing context and meaning to human emotion they generally cannot provide tools with which clinicians can examine their own work.
- Psychoanalysis may appear to be helpful in this respect, but it is very individualistic and imposes its own analytic framework at the expense of examining and analysing how ordinary clinical jobs get done.
- Interpretive social science and particularly ethnography and discourse analysis have the potential to provide the detailed descriptions of mundane practice that practitioners need to develop their capacity for 'reflection-on-and-in-action'.
- Conversation, discourse and narrative analysis can provide devices to analyse talk as text and look at how persuasive accounts are assembled and how ambiguous signs, symptoms and competing accounts are interpreted and transformed in clinicians' talk.

PART 2
Being Realistic about Clinical Judgement: Case Formulation in Context

4 Clinical science as social practice
Using formal knowledge in professional work

> Evidence does not speak for itself, but must be spoken for, and the skilled use of devices, such as personal experience and appeals to common sense, is needed to establish its relevance and credibility.
>
> (Green 2000: 473)

In this chapter, we explore the ways in which various kinds of formal knowledge are used by clinicians in the processes of case formulation, categorization and diagnosis. We challenge the popular idea of knowledge as an 'off the shelf' commodity to be selected and applied straightforwardly to cases. As Green notes above, what counts as evidence is actively negotiated in talk and interaction in a variety of settings. In current policy initiatives, there is a steadfast assumption that science delivers certainty in clinical practice. This relies on a version of science as fixed and stable, but work in philosophy and the social studies of science has problematized this idea. What serves as knowledge and truth, or as a plausible causal account, is affected by a number of processes. We begin by considering some of the processes taking place in the contexts in which science and formal knowledge are created and distributed. In particular, we consider how understandings may shift over time and what happens when formal knowledge moves away from its sites of production and into handbooks, protocols and textbooks of various kinds. The chapter then presents empirical work illustrating the use of formal knowledge in professional practice in a variety of contexts. We begin our illustrations in the more conventionally scientific domain of biomedicine and move on to consider the professions that rely on more theoretical formal knowledge, like therapeutics and social care.

From laboratory to clinic: producing and distributing science

The idea that science, or what counts as scientific fact, is in some way socially mediated is in many respects well established. The work of the influential philosopher of science Thomas Kuhn (*inter alia* 1970, 1993) may be familiar to many readers. Kuhn sought to account for the processes of conceptual change in science. He conceived of science in terms of 'paradigms', or ways of thinking that, in any one historical period, are associated with 'normal science'. These are supported by paradigm-specific concepts. He saw scientific change in terms of 'revolutions', or major shifts in ways of thinking, which Hacking describes as follows:

> Normal science ... proceeds in a rather inevitable way. Certain problems are set up, certain ways for solving them are established. What works is determined by the way the world collaborates or resists. A few anomalies are bound to persist, eventually throwing science into a crisis, followed by a new revolution.
>
> (Hacking 1999: 97)

For putting thinking in its historical context, Kuhn is widely proclaimed as one of the pioneers in the social study of science. Yet, as Hacking (1999) notes, he had very little to say about social interaction and its role in the production of either paradigms or revolutions.

The microbiologist and philosopher of science Ludwik Fleck, who wrote originally in the 1930s, has explored these social processes more comprehensively. For Fleck, the understandings held by the members of a collective (thought collective) are structured by a 'thought style'. So in scientific collectives the thought style structures ideas about what can, or should, be considered a scientific problem and about how the problem should be investigated, or dealt with. Fleck was concerned with the processes of transmission of thought styles and the ways in which the tentative science of the laboratory becomes transformed into something apparently much more stable and certain. With his emphasis on communication and language, Fleck can help us to see what happens to science as it is disseminated. He sought to understand how science changes as it moves from the 'esoteric' domains of the laboratory, into more applied settings and finally into 'popular' or 'exoteric' domains. He investigated this empirically, by analysing the structure of scientific literature, which he subclassified as 'journal', 'handbook' (**vade mecum**) or 'textbook' science (Fleck 1979: 111–12). Fleck pointed to the very social way in which laboratory science becomes gradually transformed and simplified as it becomes popularized.

'Journal science' is tentative and provisional, characterized by forms of expression, such as 'it appears possible that . . .', which invite the collective to adjudicate on the rightness or wrongness of the claims. While knowledge remains in the realm of journal science, it is available to be questioned even by relative novices in a field. In the following extract, taken from White's ethnographic study of paediatrics, a group of medical students, a registrar and a consultant are discussing the controversial theory that autism is caused by a deficiency in a metabolic hormone, secretin. The theory gained some currency in the late 1990s, mainly in the USA, leading to an increasingly vocal parents' lobby in the UK demanding the treatment.

Extract 4.1

Student 1: If I had a child with autism I would want to try it. People say it works miracles.

Reg: David's [consultant] got one [a case] from America and he says it has no effect whatsoever.

Student 2: Paul's [another consultant] doing a – what kind of trial? n = 1? He's alternating secretin and saline. Six weeks apart. They've given saline and parents say he's much better, so I don't know what he'll do. Saline is cheaper than secretin.

Cons: What? He's doing what? But we don't know how long secretin works for if it works. Do you see?

Student 2: Oh yeah, if it works for more than six weeks you wouldn't know anyway. It could be the effect of the secretin given earlier.

Cons: Exactly. This poor guy in America just wrote up some observations on three cases where he'd used secretin for gastro-intestinal things and thought he'd seen an effect and now there's all this stuff on the internet saying this or that person is doing clinical trials and when you phone them they're not. With the internet, parents are demanding it and there's absolutely no evidence.

Here, students and senior clinicians are displaying scepticism and engaging in debate, not only about the status of the claims, but about how they may properly be investigated. This is the kind of rigorous scepticism that any policy-maker would welcome, as long as the knowledge remains in the disputed realm of journal science.

However, Fleck argues that over time journal science is moulded into a simplified form via vade mecum (or handbook) science, which results from the migration of ideas through the collective. Vade mecum literally translated from the Latin means 'go with me'. In English, however, it has come to mean the kind of 'take-away knowledge', or 'knowledge to go' we find in handbooks or reference aids. The knowledge of the vade mecum is not simply a distillation of journal science, which is often characterized by contradictory claims.

Instead the vade mecum selects and assembles artefacts from journal science. Once assembled, this new, more certain science appears axiomatic and thereby has the potential to constrain thinking. Fleck notes:

> If a fact is taken to mean something fixed and proven, it exists only in vade-mecum science. The preliminary stage of disjointed signals of resistance within journal science really constitutes only the predisposition for a fact. Later, at the stage of popular knowledge, the fact becomes incarnated as an immediately perceptible object of reality.
>
> (Fleck 1979: 124–5)

This process of stabilization and predictability happens in reverse when students of science progress from the relative certainty of undergraduate studies to the unpredictability of doctoral work. Delamont and Atkinson (2001: 87), in their research into professional socialization of scientists, note:

> As undergraduates, young scientists have experienced success in their practical work because they are exposed to stage-managed experiments, demonstrations or similarly controlled environments. They encounter a world of stable and predictable phenomena under controlled conditions. In contrast, each generation or cohort of graduates has to learn that everyday research in the field of the laboratory does not necessarily produce stable, usable results until they have mastered tacit craft skills. In turn they then learn to remove all mention of those tacit, indeterminate aspects from public accounts of their research.

As handbook science travels further away from its sites of production via the media into the domain of popular science its status becomes even more simplified and 'certain'. Popular science is characterized by the omission of detail and crucially of dissenting or controversial opinion. This transforms knowledge into something 'Simplified, lucid, and apodictic' (Fleck 1979: 112). It is this apodictic knowledge that appeals to policy-makers, but it is only when science has travelled far from its sites of production that it is amenable to the simplification necessary for incorporation into protocols and guidelines.

It is tempting to think that the journey from journal to handbook to popular science takes place on a survival of the fittest basis. The best ideas thrive and are available to be disseminated in pared-down, user-friendly form. This is obviously an important part of the story. However, the potential for current handbook knowledge to limit what can plausibly be claimed means the process is a good deal more contingent than that. We can illustrate this with an example. Paul Thagard's case study of the development and acceptance of the theory that peptic ulcers are primarily caused by a bacterium, *Helicobacter pylori*, illustrates how a complex range of activities, processes and events affects the production and acceptance of new discoveries and ideas. For Thagard, scientific discovery is the product of the concatenation of individual creativity and cognition, serendipity, physical actions (like conducting an experiment), the availability of suitable technologies (such as scientific instruments) and collaborative social processes. The hypothesis, generated during the mid-1980s, that gastric ulcers were the result of bacterial infection was initially considered preposterous. The established belief at the time was that peptic ulcers were caused by excess acidity, which eventually eroded the stomach wall and caused lesions. Due to this established belief, the new hypothesis was slow to gain acceptance and was resisted both by other scientists and by clinicians. This is despite the rigour with which experiments were conducted by Warren, the pathologist who first noticed the spiral bacteria in a biopsy specimen, and Marshall, the gastroenterologist with whom he collaborated. It was not until the mid-1990s that the idea gained widespread acceptance. This depended, as Thagard notes, on a number of factors:

> The development of the bacterial theory of ulcers depended on the physical use of instruments such as microscopes and endoscopes and on the devising of experiments to test the association of *H. pylori* and gastric problems. It also had important social dimensions, including the collaborative work of Marshall, Warren and their associates; the processes of communication by which the new concepts and hypotheses spread; and the processes of negotiation by which new consensus began to form.
>
> (Thagard 1999: 39)

Thus, until Warren and Marshall's discovery of the role of *H. pylori* had entered the vade mecum it remained contested and fragile, but its entry into the vade mecum was initially blocked by the constraints imposed on thinking by the popularized 'excess acidity' explanation. So there is a good deal more to science than getting the experiments right. At their sites of production, results of experiments or observations of phenomena are interpreted and judged, and these interpretations and judgements will themselves be evaluated in different times and spaces. This interpretive work is not necessarily a solitary activity, but frequently depends on dialogue, persuasion and argument. Obviously, discussions take place in the context of a material world. We are not suggesting that all outcomes are equally valid, or that all discoveries are in some trivial way socially constructed (although, as we have said, they are socially mediated). Instead, we are suggesting that what is considered at any one time to be 'the truth' is the outcome of the diverse range of activities and contexts

Thagard outlines. EBP tends to present 'science' and formal knowledge as a straightforward solution to the problems of clinical judgement. We argue below that science and how it is made and subsequently used in practice demand investigation in their own right.

In seeking to understand how clinicians use knowledge and science, we need to be aware of the different forms of science Fleck outlines. We must see clinical encounters themselves as domains in which facts are made and assembled over time. We may thus attend to how professionals mark certainty or uncertainty in relation to the knowledge they use and examine how certainty emerges over time and space. What kinds of knowledge work as warrants for decision-making? If we take Fleck's ideas seriously, we may begin to question the idea, dominant in the literature on clinical judgement, that practice is riddled with uncertainty. We shall show below that, like scientists, professionals rely a good deal on exoteric, popular knowledge in making their judgements. If judgements depend extensively on a combination of vade mecum science and popular wisdom, we may find that professionals are often actually very good at carving certainty from ambiguity (Atkinson 1995). Thus, professional work may be seen as a complex mixture of uncertainty created by the difficulties associated with interpretation of unusual or ambiguous phenomena, or the intrinsic complexity of human relationships, and relative certainty provided by popular exoteric knowledge.

Looking and learning? Observation in practice

We begin our examination of clinical judgement in context by considering the process of observation. In the quotation below, Fleck argues that the apparently objective activities intrinsic to the scientific method, such as 'observation' or experiment, are rather more complex than they may appear:

> Observation and experiment are subject to a very popular myth. The knower is seen as a kind of conquerer, like Julius Caesar winning his battles according to the formula 'I came, I saw, I conquered'. A person wants to know something, so he makes his observation or experiment and then he knows ... But the situation is not so simple, except in certain very limited fields, such as present-day mechanics, in which there are very ancient and widely known everyday facts to draw upon. In more modern, more remote, and still complicated fields, in which it is important first to learn to observe and ask questions properly, this situation does not obtain ... until tradition, education and familiarity have produced a readiness for stylized ... perception and action; until an answer becomes largely pre-formed

in the question, and a decision is confined merely to 'yes', or 'no', or perhaps to a numerical determination; until methods and apparatus automatically carry out the greatest part of our mental work for us.

(Fleck 1979: 84)

Of course, in many clinical encounters, observation is unproblematic. Remember the idea of 'pattern recognition' discussed in Chapter 1: 'I know this is chicken pox, because I see it and recognize it.' However, in other situations observations are difficult and contested. Indeed, as Fleck notes, it seems that the more conventionally scientific domains of professional activity, in which esoteric knowledge is used, are frequently characterized by a high degree of uncertainty and equivocation. In contrast, apparently more unsettled arenas, like social care or therapeutics, where one would imagine that the range of possible interpretations of observations would increase, are often characterized by the certainty provided by popular exoteric knowledge. These settings are considered later in the chapter.

Reading and interpreting the body: Journal science in action?

We have noted that it is often in reading the artefacts of some of the most sophisticated technologies of biomedicine that interpretive difficulties occur. For example, problems have been noted in relation to the interpretation of X-rays (Pasveer 1989), echocardiographs (Daly 1989) and laboratory slides in histology, haematology and pathology (Atkinson 1995). In the context of haematology, Atkinson reminds us that the apparently neutral technical language of the laboratory in practice requires that the observer select from a vast range of available descriptions to account for what they see. That is, to do the work of diagnosis, the descriptions of the cells under the microscope are actively selected and negotiated in the talk. Of course, the cells themselves do not change, but how they are classified is subject to negotiation in interaction. As Atkinson notes, the work of the haematology department depends on:

> The identification of distinctive features, such as clefts or notches, in the samples of bone marrow or blood cells is one major task for the clinical pathologist or clinical haematologist. The observer needs to be able to characterize sizes, shapes, colours, degree of symmetry, texture and internal morphology of cells.

(Atkinson 1995: 71)

In the following extract, a discussion is taking place between two haematologists (an attending and a fellow – attending physicians are equivalent in status to a UK consultant and a fellow is roughly equivalent to a registrar) and a pathologist who has been asked for an opinion.

Extract 4.2a

F: [to pathologist] Yeah, there weren't that much then when we went back and looked we were more impressed with it, so it would be good if you could review it and see if it is atypical

At: Because the thing is that we were noticing, you know, when you see the Wright stain of the lymphocytes, quite often the cleft is right down straight and deep, right through the middle.

P: Yeah

At: Well a lot of these cleftings looked more like circumferential cleftings

P: Mm

Later in the discussion the group, accompanied by a student, look down the microscope. They are all looking at the same slide but apparently 'seeing' different things, which in turn carry different meanings for patient treatment.

Extract 4.2b

At: Those are the clefts. There's a cleft

P: A *notch*

F: Hahehh

St: Hehnhnhum huhuhm

P: Well I'd hate to have to make [a diagnosis] on this. I think the *bone marrow's* very suspicious

At: Well there *were* some there

(Atkinson 1995: 71)

Here, the pathologist is questioning both the reading of the cells and the adequacy of the sample. The discussion continues:

Extract 4.2c

At: We will try and find you another node

P: Only if you can find yourself another pathologist! [*Laughter*]

F: If you don't like it we'll change it.

P: But I don't think anybody could get around this node. It's full of germinal centres.

At: The nodules of nodular lymphoma would be bigger than that?

P: Well, no they would be this size, but they don't have this very nice mix of cell types with a lot of mitosis [cell division]

At: Mitosis suggests reactivity, do you reckon on that?

P: Yeah, I mean, that's *soft* but the highly mitotic rate tends to suggest
     reactivity . . .

(Atkinson 1995: 72)

Atkinson notes that, through exchanges such as this, the haematologists
and pathologist negotiate a mutually acceptable version of what they each see.
He also notes that there is a personal element to these negotiations, in that the
opinion of the particular pathologist involved in this case was especially
revered. Her adjudication on cases was treated as the definitive reading,
suggesting that she was believed to 'possess a personal "gift" or "eye" for
recognition and diagnosis' (Atkinson 1995: 73). This personal element can be
very important in resolving ambiguity in clinical work.

Sometimes it proves impossible to reach an agreement on what is seen.
The following extracts, from a paediatric setting, are taken from the medical
notes of an eight-month-old baby, Joanne, who presented at the accident
and emergency department with an injury to her right leg. The paediatrician
examining the child and her X-rays on admission was of the opinion that
the leg was fractured. Further, he was unconvinced by the mother's account
of the circumstances of the injury and had raised concerns that the child
may have sustained a non-accidental injury. His entry in notes reads as
follows:

Extract 4.3a
Discussed with radiologists. Skeletal survey films show what is
generally agreed to be mid-shaft fracture of right femur undisplaced.
No periosteal reaction. There is a query regarding a small fracture of left distal metaphysis [growing portion] of femur. I have
explained all this to mother and said that we may need further
opinions. Discussed with [consultant paediatric radiologist at
regional children's hospital] send X-rays, originals not copies by taxi
for his opinion.

Here the paediatrician explicitly refers to the need to ensure that he and the
consultant radiologist are looking at the same thing ('original not copies'). The
report of the consultant radiologist states:

Extract 4.3b
I have now reviewed this child's radiographs. The initial right femur
film does show a linear (illegible word) extending obliquely across
the mid-shaft of the femur, but this is not convincing for a fracture
and is not seen on a later film. There is a small apparent fragment
continuous with the posterior margin of the left distal femoral
and metaphysis. I cannot exclude a metaphysial fracture here, but

considerable irregularity may be seen here normally. No other fracture seen. If clinically warranted, repeat films in 1–2 weeks should show callous formation if there is a fracture . . . The present films are unconvincing.

The expert opinion expressed here is considerably more tentative than the paediatrician's. The account is coded in the tentative language of journal science; for example, 'this is *not convincing* for a fracture', 'I *cannot exclude* a metaphysial fracture here'. The report illustrates a frequent problem in the interpretation of test results. It is often difficult to distinguish between 'normal' variation and the presence of disease or injury, and it is senior clinicians who appear most likely to raise these doubts. In response, the X-rays were repeated and reviewed by a specialist registrar in orthopaedics, who wrote:

Extract 4.3c
Fresh X-rays have been done today which show that there was frank callous formation over the mid-shaft of the femur and there was an old fracture there. This has healed without any problems and is in perfect position.

The selection of the words 'show', 'there was', 'has healed' code this account as 'fact', not opinion. However, again, the consultant orthopaedic surgeon interprets the X-rays differently:

Extract 4.3d
Diagnosis of right femoral fracture was based on the history of thigh swelling and tenderness and the equivocal X-ray appearance. I risk the various radiologists' opinions and argue that the diagnosis of fracture is uncertain. I do not think there is a significant injury on the left side . . . I think that a bone scan should be done but may be over-investigating. I would be grateful for the paediatrician's view on this. Will see at fracture clinic in 3/52 with further X-ray right femur.

This account from the senior clinician illustrates the more tentative and uncertain language of journal science. Throughout the accounts above, there are questions raised that cannot be answered entirely by recourse to science or objective criteria. For example, the consultant radiologist suggests that the X-rays be repeated 'if clinically warranted', and the orthopaedic surgeon suggests that a bone scan may be 'over-investigating'. In short, even decisions to investigate require something more than reasoning by numbers. The essentially ethical or moral decision about whether to use radioactive material in further investigations is deferred to the paediatrician, who justifies his decision to proceed with an isotope bone scan as follows:

Extract 4.3e
Orthopaedic comments noted, I think an isotope bone scan will be needed because of:

1 Medico-legal
2 Controversial X-ray reports

An isotope bone scan was duly undertaken, with the following results:

Extract 4.3f
Abnormalities present within the right femur. On the initial blood pool study there is evidence of a little increased uptake within the mid-shaft of the right femur. On the later static images there is small area of focal increased uptake within the mid-shaft with more diffuse increased uptake extending towards both epiphyses, but particularly the lower one. The appearances are obviously non-specific and will be in keeping for example with trauma or infection. However the mid-shaft location is perhaps more in keeping with a fracture. No definite focal area of increased uptake can be identified.

Following extensive investigations, the information obtained remains uncertain and equivocal. The facts in the isotope bone scan are clear ('there is small area of focal increased uptake within the mid-shaft with more diffuse increased uptake extending towards both epiphyses, but particularly the lower one'), but the opinion is not ('The appearances are obviously non-specific and will be in keeping for example with trauma or infection'). The bone scan cannot interpret itself. Neither, in this case, can it provide clear answers to feed the process of clinical judgement. As this case potentially involved a child at risk, failure to reach some kind of decision was unacceptable. Professionals had to act, and in so doing had to rely on other kinds of knowledge and reasoning, such as their judgements about the veracity of the parents' story and their evaluation of the parental relationship with Joanne.

The examples above show how potentially contestable are the artefacts of technological medicine. In one sense, this seems to be a rather alarming and counterintuitive observation. Technology is supposed to reduce diagnostic uncertainty. Yet the interpretive problems we have illustrated are entirely consistent with Fleck's notion of journal science. The more esoteric the knowledge, the more likely it is to produce equivocal formulations. Indeed, questioning the status of knowledge is one of the ways in which clinicians may display their expertise. This tendency can be seen most markedly when understandings remain in the realm of journal science; that is, before they have been accepted as valid by a thought collective, as we saw in the secretin example above. However, it is not uncommon for experienced clinicians to question the more stable vade mecum science. In fact, resurrecting the more tentative voice of journal science may be an important way in which practitioners display their competence. Thus, exposure to clinical practice may form an intermediate point in which novices have their handbook knowledge destablized by more experienced professionals.

This sceptical approach is illustrated in the following two extracts taken from pre-clinic briefing sessions between a consultant and a registrar.

Extract 4.4

Con: He's been in with asthma but that's not why he comes to see us (.4). The main reason is some hydronephrosis – I think I've got the last [ct?] – seems to have a problem attending [reading] Repeat ultrasound October 99, it's still hydronephrosis, further up (.5) urinary tract infection, yeah, for definite.

Reg: That's back in (.) April

Con: Back in April. DMSA [dimercaptosuccinic acid – test to assess scarring and relative function of kidney] clear. Mild right sided hydronephrosis with prominent renal pelvis mainly extra renal, no scarring and (.) no (.) reflux. (.7) So, I suppose I thought that the best way was to do repeat the ultrasound if the kidney was blowing up and we needed a (), so that's fine. It's difficult sometimes with these mild hydronephrosis. You never know whether it's the beginning of –

Reg: Or whether it's borderline –

Con: Or whether it's just the [way] they're made –

Reg: [Yeah] yeah

The consultant's account has a number of markers of certainty ('urinary tract infection, yeah, for definite') but these are juxtaposed with markers of uncertainty, warranted principally by clinical experience ('It's difficult some-times with these mild hydronephrosis'), accompanied by references to the limits and fallibility of the technology. The difficulty in adjudicating between the normal and pathological is explicitly stated.

In the following exchange, clinicians are discussing two children from the same extended family who both have cerebral palsy (CP). The clinicians are contesting the status of the diagnostic category 'birth asphyxia', which was thought, until the late 1980s, to be the principal aetiology of CP, and therefore was firmly established in the vade mecum of that time.

Extract 4.5

Con: . . . Daisy was born at term and for no reason whatsoever started to have seizures in the neonatal period and ended up heavily sedated and ventilated –

Reg: Ooooer

Con: – No reason found for her seizures and (.7) you know assumed birth as –, whatever birth asphyxia is.

Reg: Yeah rather a dubious term

Con: Yeah – hhh, non-entity term, well she illustrates it well really, erm and now has cerebral palsy, erm not under my care . . . This [other] child was born in exactly the same thing, severe seizure disorder, lots of anticonvulsants, but is mobile now, athetoid movements bowel problems, with erm excess salivation, some fits. Erm, both subsequent children, each family's had a subsequent child which was monitored for 24 hours on special care erm, immediately after extraction by Caesarian section and didn't fit at all.

Reg: I see

Con: So it's bizarre and the geneticists can't actually find a diagnosis, or a particular link between them and they've actually ended up with different patterns of cerebral palsy. So it's bizarre . . .

Clearly, this child did not have seizures 'for no reason whatsoever', but in using this phrase the consultant references the limits of currently available knowledge. She stops herself mid-word, to display her knowledge that 'birth asphyxia' is a problematic category, which is immediately affirmed by the registrar. The consultant's story of both children developing 'unexplained' seizures from birth has a dual function. First, it is being used to engage with the registrar in a mutual display of their competence, as they join in gently mocking the vade mecum of a 'previous era'. The consultant then moves to display her competence in relation to the 'new' vade mecum – the genetics of CP. Thus, in this context, the registar's rather knowing 'I see' and the consultant's repeated 'So it's bizarre' can be heard as surprise (and disappointment) – given the family history – that the case doesn't corroborate the 'new' vade mecum.

There are some interesting contextual matters relating to this extract. The birth asphyxia hypothesis has been used extensively in claims for compensation in cases involving an infant developing CP following a normal delivery, where there had been a degree of foetal distress during labour. Mild foetal distress is very common and does not necessarily indicate the need for a Caesarian section. Thus, if an obstetrician decides against surgery, but the child subsequently develops CP, the doctor risks their actions being judged retrospectively as medical error. The genetic hypothesis is a major challenge to these kinds of cases and is one way in which neonatal paediatricians can display their solidarity with their obstetric colleagues in this potentially litigious domain. It may also have accelerated the passage of the genetic hypothesis into the vade mecum. Thus, 'science talk' in clinical contexts may also do important cultural and moral work. We consider these matters further in Chapter 5.

The equivocations associated with science are often accompanied by anecdotes, which function as homilies or fables pointing to the right course of action. Unlike the tentative journal science mode, these anecdotes are coded as reliable and factual. In the following exchange, taken from Atkinson's study, a student, an attending and a fellow are discussing problems related to the use of heparin (an anticoagulant). They are talking about a patient who as a result of a 'heparin induced state' had suffered an amputation. The patient's problems were therefore largely iatrogenic (caused by medicine), which is a tricky moral domain. The doctors are discussing the potential costs and benefits of another drug, protamine, which is sometimes used to neutralize heparin in situations where patients are considered to be at risk of haemorrhage.

Extract 4.6a

St: Does heparin have a pretty short half life, doesn't it? So

F: Yeah, but there is a certain . . . there's a certain amount I think that *does* get bound to the platelet and the endothelium and sticks around. In most cases *stopping* it or starting aspirin, and there's been a suggestion the reason why protamine hasn't and it's been sort of *twofold*. One they're not sure exactly what they're neutralizing, and two they feel that they may *exacerbate* the problem with the protamine. Since you have somebody who's *clotting* and to give them *pro*tamine, you know as Dr de Kalb says, you don't *titrate* it right, who knows how to *titrate* it, then you might actually make things *worse*

(Adapted from Atkinson 1995: 137)

The fellow's account shows characteristic markers of uncertainty associated with the voice of journal science. At this point the attending physician interjects and asks, 'You got time for a quick anecdote?' He proceeds to tell a story about another 'heparin-induced' case, which led to a stroke and ultimately the death of a famous movie star. The attending uses the 'voice of personal experience' (Atkinson 1995: 139), as we can see in the following edited extract:

Extract 4.6b

A: . . . There she was and there was blood in the spinal fluid. I drew blood from her and started doing a *clot*ting time and you know sort of (inverting) it in there, the blood wouldn't clot.

F: Mhuh

A: And I stood there for forty-five minutes and an hour and it wouldn't *clot.* So I had some of my *own* blood taken and we mixed *my* blood with *her* blood and then *my* blood wouldn't clot. So she had some sort of, certainly, anticoagulant, and it was really severe, because when I diluted her blood it *still* had anticoagulant

F: Mm

A: I *then* found that she'd been going to an internist in Beverly Hills who was giving people *heparin* in large doses to prevent atherosclerosis or something . . . And er I got out the protamine and I tried to *tit*rate it used a little bit in vitro before giving it to her and calculated a *dose*, and we gave it to her and then I was supposed to come back the next day for re*peat* tests and as I was driving down Sunset Boulevard I had my radio on and I heard she'd died.

(Atkinson 1995: 138)

This anecdote is not a distraction from the process of case formulation, it is integral to the discussions. The first-hand account carries considerable evidential weight in contrast to the tentative coding of the fellow's scientific account. It also has the moral effect of reinforcing the fellow's earlier warning that 'you might actually make things worse'. So, far from being 'purely anecdotal', anecdotes transmit clinical maxims that draw upon and augment practitioners' formal knowledge.

In summary, this section has argued that the more technological areas of clinical practice are often the most uncertain. However, we should not exaggerate this phenomenon. There are many occasions on which test results of various kinds are treated as warrants for certainty. For example, in a study we consider in more detail in Chapter 5, Anspach found that in life and death prognostic decision-making in a neonatal unit, technological cues, such as respirator settings, blood gases and electrolyes, were treated by physicians as more reliable than interactive cues, such as responsiveness, reported by the nurses (Anspach 1987). So it would be folly to argue that science in some straightforward way equals uncertainty. Indeed, when combined with the 'voice of personal experience' it may well provide a feeling of certainty, or rather a sense of the 'correctness' of our actions. However, we *have* sought to trouble the popular view that science necessarily equals certainty. As part of that exoteric domain of popular knowledge, this presumption is now largely unquestioned by the public and by policy-makers. Yet it is perhaps by operating with the scepticism of journal science and all its attendent uncertainty that clinicians are at their best, since scepticism requires effort and thought. But there is also much professional activity that must take place in the territory of popular knowledge. If Fleck is correct, we would expect this to provide the domains of relative certainty in clinical judgement.

Beyond 'knowledge to go?' Popular knowledge and clinical practice

> There are many contexts in which uncertainty is not an issue for the actors, because they employ practical reasoning and action in such a way as to produce relatively unproblematic diagnoses and disposals . . . personal knowledge and experience are not normally treated by practitioners as reflections of uncertainty, but as warrants for certainty. The primacy of direct experience, for instance, is taken to guarantee knowledge which the student or practitioner can *rely* on.
>
> (Atkinson 1995: 114–15)

In the quotation above, Atkinson warns against the reductionist use of the concept of uncertainty and reminds us that much clinical activity is undertaken with apparent certainty, or even dogmatism (Bosk 1979). We have already noted Fleck's argument that, however specialized our field, a major portion of the knowledge we use is in the domain of popular science, or knowledge for non-experts. This is particularly the case where judgements about people, relationships and personality are a central feature of the work, where practitioners rely substantially on practical–moral reasoning. We have more to say about the moral dimensions of this in Chapter 5. However, here we want to illustrate how, in contrast to the voice of journal science, these judgements tend to operate as warrants for certainty in clinical judgement. Presented below is a letter from a child psychiatrist to a consultant paediatrician concerning a teenage boy, Paul.

Extract 4.7

Dear Dr Dhokia,

Thank you for asking me to see Paul. It was revealing that both father and son have a similar temperament and during the interview with Paul, father commented he was worried Paul would not cooperate with me. In fact father seemed almost to pre-empt Paul's fears and in that way encourage them. During the interview Paul drew a picture of his father and a picture of himself looking worried. Paul said he was worried about father and also worried about other children at school. It seems therefore that Paul presents with an anxiety state with evidence of aggression and that he now fears going to school. Possibly precipitated by intercurrent illness, i.e. chicken pox three weeks ago. It seems that Paul has a difficult personality and that he has always been sensitive and anxious and was in fact a difficult baby following a Keelans forceps birth. Father too becomes anxious and sensitive – an example is given above in this letter. Mother was reassured by the explanation of these problems but father found it difficult to be reassured and this may contribute to further difficulties helping him settle back in school.

I suppose a differential diagnosis here would be a post-encephalitic state, although there is no complaint of headache and no neurological signs. However I undertook to see the family again and if the problems persist I could check his EEG providing it is not too long after his original chicken pox. Reassurance and advice on handling with his graded reintroduction to school, limit setting but sympathy for his anxiety, help mother and I think father was relieved to be able to discuss the problem openly. Because of this I have offered to see them again for follow up to see how things are going. It seems worthwhile to have them seen quickly to hopefully prevent the problem getting chronic.

The psychiatrist's report has a dogmatic and certain flavour. He talks of the boy's and his father's temperaments being 'revealed' to him. His formulation is that both father and son are 'worriers', and this explains Paul's problems at home and school. The direct observations of the interactions between father and son are read as reliable signs of a fixed and enduring pattern of family relations. This primary formulation is used to interpret the boy's drawing and to decide on treatment and disposal. Although we can see some limited use of psychiatric discourse – for example, 'anxiety state' – this formulation relies substantially on exoteric knowledge. It is only when the psychiatrist mentions the possible differential diagnosis 'post-encephalic state' that any tentativeness or equivocation is shown.

It is judgements like this about people and personalities that often have an apodictic flavour in professionals' talk. The formulations in these circumstances rely substantially on moral categorization and characterizations of the patient or client and their significant others. In many settings, this kind of moral work sits alongside more formal scientific reasoning. We will not say very much more about this here, as Chapter 5 is specifically oriented to the moral aspects of practice. We also provide an extended example from a paediatric setting in Chapter 6, which shows some of the ways in which different kinds of reasoning are brought together to do the work of case formulation. Having explored the use of formal knowledge in biomedicine, we now need to consider the domain of human relationships and the impact of various psychological theories upon practice.

Reading relationships: psychological theory and observation

> And then I see it, altogether, in one pure thought bite; the Quantity Theory of Insanity shows its face to me. I suppose all people who look for the first time upon some new, large scale, explanatory theory must feel as I did at that moment. With one surge of tremendous arrogance, of aching hubris, I felt as if I were looking at the very form of whatever purpose, whatever explanation, there really is inherent in the very stuff of this earth, this life . . . 'What if . . .' I thought to myself, 'What if there is only a fixed proportion of sanity available in any given society at any given time?' . . . For years I had sought some hypothesis to cement the individual psyche to the group; it was right in front of me all the time. But I went on, I elaborated, I filled out the theory, or rather it filled out itself. It fizzed and took on form the way a paper flower expands in water.
>
> (Self 1994: 126)

The above quote is taken from Will Self's satirical novel about psychiatry. Like all satire, it exaggerates and amplifies, but it relies for its power on the recognizability of its subject matter. If it is too far removed from what we think we know, satire ceases to be funny. Thus, Will Self is making a serious point about the effect that theory has on our perception of reality and about theory's capacity to feed itself. We have said that professions concerned with human relationships and emotion rely to a large extent on exoteric, practical–moral reasoning. However, we must consider the effect of theory, specifically psychological theory, on such reasoning. While many commentators have noted that in the murkier areas of professional practice like social work, or therapeutic services, practitioners make very little explicit use of theory (for example, Stevenson and Parsloe 1978; Potter 1982; John 1990), we show below that the implicit and explicit use of psychological theory is one of the principal ways in which practitioners warrant their case formulations. Theoretical knowledge is very different from journal science. Rather as Will Self describes, it operates much like handbook science in that it reduces uncertainty in particular kinds of ways:

1 Theory operates like a powerful lens and has a marked effect on observation and hence on what counts as a fact, as we show below.

2 Just as journal science is simplified as it passes into more popular domains, so too is psychological theory (Burman 1990, 1994; White, 1998). This is evident in the vast numbers of schedules and checklists of child development, psychological health and social

adjustment used routinely by social workers, nurses and other professionals.

3 Psychological theory is easily popularized. Once it enters popular wisdom we may expect it to be treated as trivially true. It can thus be used as a highly flexible resource to warrant moral judgements (White 2001).

Let us examine what the implications of this are for the processes of case formulation. Case formulation relies substantially on observation. We have already raised some questions about observation in biomedical settings using Ludwik Fleck's ideas, but how do these translate to the observation of human relationships? It will helpful if we illustrate our arguments with an example. The following quote is taken from a highly respected text on the psychological and psychiatric assessment of parenting (Reder and Lucey 1995). It is referring to expert assessments conducted as part of legal proceedings.

> The role of the expert assessor in advising the legal process is to draw together information based upon a general knowledge of child development, theoretical frameworks that are informed by research and academic understanding and the particular circumstances of the child in question so that an opinion is available which is a synthesis of these components.
>
> (Baker 1995: 248)

This would appear at first sight to be a fairly uncontroversial statement about the role of the 'expert assessor' in situations where there is concern about parent–child relationships. It conjures up an image of the rational, independent expert - with privileged access to the clear, undisputed 'circumstances' of the case on one side and the incontrovertible, apodictic truth of formal systems of knowledge on the other – making objective judgements informed by hard theory and empirical evidence.

Now, we want you to imagine this scenario: you have been asked to observe the relationship between a three-year-old child and his father, with a view to deciding whether the father should be allowed to have the child come to stay with him each week. The child arrives tearful, distressed and clinging to his mother. The father appears embarrassed and becomes slightly irritated with the child and the mother. He protests to you that this has never happened on previous contacts. All his somewhat clumsy efforts to comfort the child are rejected and only seem to increase the child's distress and anger the mother. The mother looks at you fleetingly with an 'I told you so' expression. How would you make sense of these events? How would you impose some sort of order on this fast flowing sequence of interaction? In imposing some sort of order, what inferences do we make about the dispositions and characters of the participants and their relationships?

To do this ordering work, it is very likely that we would invoke some article of formal knowledge. Much of the research in the field of 'good' parenting has been carried out from a social learning theory perspective. This posits that one of the main influences on child behaviour is the overt behaviour of parents and other family members. Consequently, particular importance is placed on the micro-interaction: the moment-by-moment patterns and processes within parent–child interaction. From this theoretical perspective, these micro-observations are predictive of 'good' parent–child relationships. Hence these approaches have generated a cornucopia of check-lists and inventories to assist the practitioner in their observations of parents and children in interaction; to help them break down the flow of interaction into more managable, discrete, operationalized components. An example of such a checklist (Herbert 1996) is given in Figure 4.1.

	Often	Occasionally	Never
Plays contentedly			
Laughs and smiles			
Runs			
Talks freely			
Comes for help			
Comes for comfort			
Cuddles up to mother or father			
Responds to affection			
Responds to attention			
At ease with parents when near him or her			
Joins in activities with siblings and friends			
Makes eye contact with parents			

Figure 4.1 The child's behaviour at home.

Obviously these observational tools have their strengths. But the problem with them is that what constitutes 'good' interaction is determined by the theoretical assumptions that underlie their production. In other words we only end up 'looking for' and 'seeing' what our theoretical lens allows us to see.

In contrast with social learning theory, the theory underlying, for example, the assessment of attachment relationships advocates that practitioners look for rather different things in their observations. This is illustrated by Figure 4.2, which is taken from Vera Fahlberg's (1979) 'attachment checklist'. This represents an example of a more 'open' observational method that encourages the observer to view and then reflect on a whole extended sequence of interaction. So the questions are mere prompts to help the observer to organize their observations of attachment behaviour. In a sense, the checklist is the embodiment of attachment theory.

A crucial difference between social learning theory and attachment theory is the status given to overt behaviour. According to attachment theory, observed behaviour (for example, a toddler avoiding his mother when reunited with her after a short separation) is used to make an inference

One to five years

Does the child:	Does the parent(s):
• explore the environment in a normal way? • respond to parent(s)? • keep occupied in a positive way? • seem relaxed and happy? • have the ability to express emotions? • react to pain and pleasure? • engage in age appropriate activity? • use speech appropriately? • express frustration? • respond to parental limit setting? • exhibit observable fears? • react positively to physical closeness? • respond appropriately to separation from parent? • respond appropriately to parent's return? • exhibit body rigidity or relaxation? Others:	• use appropriate disciplinary measures? • show interest in child's development? • respond to child's overtures? • encourage physical closeness with the child? • comfort the child in a positive way? • initiate positive interactions with the child? • accept expressions of autonomy? • see the child as 'taking after' someone? Is this positive or negative? Others:

Figure 4.2   Observation checklist: what to look for in assessing attachment.

about a covert, underlying theoretical construct, namely insecure attachment. Thus, given the different theoretical assumptions underlying social learning and attachment theory, it is possible for two observers, motivated and influenced by different theoretical models, to emerge with quite different interpretations of the same sequence of interaction.

In sum, the questionnaires, checklists, indeed all 'technologies' of assessment are the handbook embodiments of theories. As such, they can construct versions of reality and affect what we 'see' when we 'observe', as John (1990: 127) notes:

> just as theories are underdetermined by facts, so facts are over-determined by theory, which means that situations may be capable of a range of factual interpretations depending on the theory selected. Furthermore, individual psychological theories have been shown to be capable of such a degree of interpretive flexibility as to be virtually incorrigible; it has sometimes been difficult to find situations, even when they involve quite contradictory outcomes, which they could not plausibly explain.

We gave an example in Chapter 3 of the way in which psychoanalytic ideas can rewrite and reinterpret people's accounts and experiences, and other psychological theories have the same potential. In the following example, a clinical psychologist is discussing an eight-year-old child, Grace, and her mother, Dawn.

Extract 4.8
One of them is a girl called Grace Sheehan, who witnessed an assault on her mother a year and a half ago or something. Ehm and has had a traumatic reaction. I assessed them and it is clear that the mother has got quite severe PTSD [post-traumatic stress disorder] and that Grace is also traumatized, but one of the problems is that Mrs Sh–, Dawn won't speak to Grace about any of this, she won't she tries very hard to avoid all subjects and changes the subject when Grace tries to talk about it she gets very upset, Dawn gets very upset and very anxious. We talked a lot about you know maybe the best thing to do would be that I help Dawn deal with her trauma first then she's going to be in a much better position to help her daughter. Ehm they've got all the classic sort of pushing the thoughts away, keeping very busy, very very avoidant. Her life is also now avoiding places where this assault happened and lots of nightmares lots of re-experiencing ehm in the meantime you know we talked about how it was important for Grace to express herself and talk about what's happened and she now talks to other people instead of her mother.

This extract illustrates how the theory underpinning the diagnosis 'post-traumatic stress disorder' governs the way the psychologist tells the case. This account is quite different from the version given by the mother and daughter, who would not routinely use concepts like 'pushing the thoughts away', 'very very avoidant', or 're-experiencing'. The psychologist's version of the mother's attempts to 'cope' in the aftermath of the assault are constructed as 'pathological', in that 'it is clear' that they represent the signs and symptoms of 'severe PTSD'. Moreover, the mother's disorder and her inappropriate response to her daughter's need to talk about the assault are used to explain the daughter's continuing symptoms. In so doing, the psychologist invokes the knowledge of vade mecum; that is, only by repeatedly being able to talk about the original trauma will Grace and her mother find relief from their distress. Thus, this account does not simply describe a reality. It re-writes observation through the lens of theory. Of course, this is not necessarily a problem. For example, if professionals use theory self-consciously, they may juxtapose one theoretical perspective against another, which may help them to be more thoroughgoing, questioning and rigorous in their work. However, as we can see above, theory is often treated as synonymous with 'truth' and is not appoached in this critical manner. As John notes above, the problem with psychological theories is that they are potentially highly reductionist. That is, they can be used to explain anything. This is because they coalesce so easily with popular knowledge and they are thus often invoked to provide 'authoritative warrant for decisions taken on other grounds' (John 1990: 116).

This is particularly so in morally laden domains like therapy. In the extract below a team of family therapists and a social worker are discussing a therapy session.

Extract 4.9a
1   Th2: Well I felt that was one big gigantic flop (laughs)
2   Cons1: Well I think =
3   Th2: = Because I felt all the time we were sort of (2.0) it was almost a
4   real systemic thing the more we tried to be positive the more
5   accepting the more she dredged up dreadful things about herself
6   Cons1: Mm
7   Th2: About the family. And I feel there's such a strong (0.5) belief
8   Cons2: Can I ask why it took you so long to get over here?
9   Th1: Oh she collared me in the waiting room and said I want to talk
10 about it in the video room. Well is it not something you could
11 talk about standing here? No no no I want him to come into
12 hospital here for a full assessment. I want something further than
13 family therapy. I believe there is something wrong and (0.5) we
14 need to find out what it is because (0.5) she believes we aren't

15   seeing the true David
16 Cons2: Yeah in a sense that is very important 'cos that makes more
17   sense of the session to me because that makes me feel that she's
18   sort of upping the stakes =
19 Th2: = Right =
20 Cons2: = To the [extent that I just realised that we are not getting
         through =
21 Th2: [Right
22 Cons2: [= At all, because I really had to sit through =
23 Th2: [Right
24 Cons2: = It thinking it wasn't working or (are we giving the right
         structure?)
25 Cons1: [So did you
26 SW: [Grandmother thought that was a waste of the time because she
27   wasn't getting what she wanted =

Clearly, the therapist (Th2) does not feel that the session has been a success
because the grandmother in the case has resisted her attempts to reframe the
family difficulties in a positive light. This idea of reframing, or 'positive
connotation', is derived from **family systems theory**, and forms part of the
conceptual arsenal of family therapists. In her second turn Th1 uses another
concept, 'complementarity' (Watzlawick *et al.* 1967; Bateson 1978), to account
for the failure. Complementary interaction, put simply, consists of reciprocity
between participants whose actions are responses to, and elicited by, the
actions of the other, almost in an equal and opposite way. For example, an
interaction would be complementary if one party's aggressive and accusatory
outburst was met with an outpouring of apology and remorse by the other,
which in turn elicits more aggression from the first party. Thus, the grandmother's self-blame is seen as part of an escalating cycle of increasingly
determined efforts at positive connotation by the therapists being met with
equally determined efforts by the grandmother to depict herself and the
family negatively.

At line 8, the therapist's account is interrupted by her colleague, who
asks why there was such a delay in bringing the family from the waiting
room over to the interview room. Th1 (lines 9–15) then tells a story of
her encounter with grandmother in the waiting room. First, the therapist
describes herself being 'collared'; conveying a sense of the encounter being
unexpected and unwanted. She then makes use of reported speech to detail
the conversation which took place in the waiting room. This portrays
grandmother's dissatisfaction with the therapy and her belief that there is
'something wrong' with her grandson and that the team are 'not seeing the
true David' in the family meetings. Cons2 then uses the therapist's story of
grandmother's behaviour in the waiting area to make sense of the therapist's

failure to get the family to identify their strengths and achievements. She describes grandmother 'sort of upping the stakes to the extent . . . that we're not getting through at all'. At this point, the therapists appear to be making an interpretation of grandmother's storytelling in the session, viewing it as a response to their strategy of focusing on the family's strengths. However, as the discussion moves on, this formulation is displaced by a very different claim, which has consequences for grandmother's moral identity and forms the basis of the therapy team's version of the family troubles. This is illustrated in the following extract:

Extract 4.9b

SW: Yeah I think actually I spoke to grandad before I went in to see them and really what he was hinting is that she's just moaning, moaning, nagging, nagging, nagging all the time and he wants a break from that really. What's *definitely* happening is that their relationship is becoming increasingly stressed. (2.0)

Th2: I can well see that why he feels like that. There's this quality of just wanting to go on and on =

Cons2: = Sort of breast beating =

Th2: = Yes sort of breast beating. You know (1.0) and always by trying to be positive she thinks you're not hearing and that's why we didn't particularly carry on in that way. (1.5) It didn't seem to be (any use at all).

In this extract, the social worker constructs the fact that the grandparents' relationship is '*definitely* . . . increasingly stressed' and attributes this, using an **extreme case formulation** (see Glossary), to grandmother 'just moaning, moaning, nagging, nagging, nagging all the time'. This claim is based on her interpretation of a recent conversation with grandfather.

The therapist confirms the social worker's claim by relating it to her own experience of the grandmother's storytelling in the session: 'I can well see that why he feels like that. There's this quality of just wanting to go on and on.' The consultant latches on to this description and refers to grandmother 'sort of breast beating', which is immediately affirmed by the therapist, who then again makes a link between grandmother's story and the therapists' futile attempts to focus on the positive. However, as the next extract shows, the ascription of moral identity ('breast beating') is used later in the talk, when the team work up a version of the troubles that blames grandmother.

Extract 4.9c

Cons1: So would you want to feedback to them then about how (.) what you felt about the session ((*trails off*))

Cons2: I mean (.) I suppose just just to add to that. >Bit boring and down to earth< I have the sense that the story we are hearing is just mum's (.) in the fact that it goes on and on and on and on. >Well *blast* her feelings about ((her daughter))< Grandmother's just not listening to any of them and they just spend ages going round. She's got to separate that *off* (1.0) from how she gets on with Des.

Th1: It's irritating. When ((Th2)) started to talk about David she sort of blocked it off and started to talk about her.

Cons1: It does in fact have the opposite effect from what she hopes. In that if she goes on telling people people will listen and then take notice well actually it has the opposite effect doesn't it?

The extract begins with Cons1 asking the team to consider what the therapists will feed back to the family. However, at the next turn, her colleague ignores this question and makes an overt evaluation of grandmother's role in the troubles. Having referred to the unrelenting nature of grandmother's version ('the story we are hearing is just grandmother's, it goes on and on and on and on'), Cons2 is critical of grandmother and her 'breast beating' about her role in the removal of the children from her daughter ('Well *blast* her feelings about ((her daughter))'). Then she infers that grandmother is unable to hear other family members' stories and perspectives and the dialogue is unchanging because of her. ('Grandmother's just not listening to any of them and they just spend ages going round.')

In this example, systems theory, in the form of the concept of complementarity, is used rhetorically to warrant the therapists' moral judgements. First it is invoked to account for an observed interactional difficulty in a therapy session. However, this is subsequently reclassified as an enduring characteristic of the family's communication and relationships. This then becomes pivotal to the therapists' explanation of the family troubles. A formulation is constructed in which the grandmother is blamed for not listening and causing all the other family members to 'shut off'.

In the next and final extract a social worker is describing one of her clients. Here there is no explicit reference to theory, but the popular version of psychological ideas is used to produce a formulation about the case that is clear and unequivocal and forms the basis for the social worker's work.

Extract 4.10

Yes, I mean she's a very angry person but, so there are a lot of issues probably in the past that she could perhaps do with working through, whether she will or not I don't know. Her family have all turned against her because she drinks . . . In fact really if she had a more supportive family I think her problems would be a lot less, it's just that she's completely on her own with an aggressive nature. I mean, I was quite pleased today because I've had quite a few conversations with her about her aggression and how she deals with people and in the core group today I mean she started off saying she was going to kill the head teacher, she was going fucking punch her and all this sort of thing, but she was quite assertive really. She said what she had to say, not in a way that I would . . . so perhaps a bit of it's sinking in I don't know.

Here the social worker makes use of popular psychological knowledge. Her formulation draws implicitly on the ideas about early trauma associated with psychodynamic theory: 'so there are a lot of issues probably in the past that she could perhaps do with working through'. It makes explicit attributions of cause and effect ('really if she had a more supportive family I think her problems would be a lot less'), but also blames the client, or rather her drinking habits, for her not having a 'supportive family': 'her family have all turned against her because she drinks'. She uses reported speech to support her claims about the client's aggressiveness, but goes on to employ contrastive rhetoric to mark the effect of her own interventions: 'but she was quite assertive really. She said what she had to say, not in a way that I would . . . so perhaps a bit of it's sinking in I don't know.' As we would expect, this relatively popularized knowledge grants an apodictic, undisputed and irrefutable status to the formulations and enables the social worker to categorize and process the case and also to account for her actions. Moreover, because it invokes her status as eyewitness, it would be exceedingly difficult to challenge without compelling contradictory evidence.

In the relatively exoteric domain of human relationships, then, professional talk centres not so much on uncertainty, but on complex characterizations, often delivered unequivocally, with detailed stories about what has happened, who should change and how they should do so. These formulations may or may not be accompanied by references to specific theories. That is, the popular nature of the ideas invoked apparently exempts practitioners from the imperative to justify their actions using formal knowledge.

> Common sense is a powerful rhetoric because it creates a sense of shared values between speaker and audience, which is difficult to resist without explicitly rejecting these values. It is also a device which constitutes expert knowledges as redundant, simply because what is said is self-evident and known by everybody.
>
> (Green 2000: 470)

Moreover, we can see that the more popular knowledge becomes the more it accomplishes moral work. This means that we should be opening up professional 'common sense' for examination and debate. We examine the moral dimensions of practice further in the next chapter.

Summary

- We have argued that there is a need for more complex understandings of the nature and use of formal knowledge across the range of health and welfare settings.
- We have sought to trouble the idea that science always delivers certainty. In esoteric domains science may in fact increase uncertainty. This is an important message for those professionals who look to more esoteric domains to provide them with clear answers. For example, social workers in child care teams often become irritated with paediatricians when they cannot give a definitive view on whether a child's injury is the result of an accident or an assault. Yet we can see from some of the examples above that the idea that information can straightforwardly deliver answers is not always sustainable.
- We have also wanted to destabilize the equally crude idea that clinicians are always riddled with uncertainty. Handbook science, psychological theory, personal experience and popular knowledge all function as effective warrants for certainty, perhaps in those domains where hanging on to uncertainty may be a more appropriate and rigorous option.
- In seeking to subvert the dominant policy view of clinical judgement as a straightforward process of knowledge use, we do not wish to 'socialize' all decision-making. Particularly in biomedicine, diagnostic tests and technologies often form an indispensable bedrock for many clinical decisions.
- However, work in the philosophy of science and ethnographic studies can be illuminating and useful in showing precisely how science is produced and transmitted and how professionals mark certainty or uncertainty in relation to the formal knowledge that they use. By seeing knowledge in this live and complex way, we may open up for debate aspects of clinical work obscured in more normative and prescriptive studies.

5 Emotion and morality
Blameworthiness, creditworthiness and clinical judgement

> I suggest only that certain aspects of the process of emotion and feeling are indispensable for rationality. At their best, feelings point us in the proper direction, take us to the appropriate place in a decision-making space, where we may put the instruments of logic to good use. We are faced by uncertainty when we have to make a moral judgement . . . Emotion and feeling, along with the covert physiological machinery underlying them, assist us with the daunting task of predicting an uncertain future and planning our actions accordingly.
>
> (Damasio 1994: xiv–xv)

In Chapter 4 we showed how handbook and popular versions of knowledge or theory can be used to justify case formulations, many of which perform important moral work. In this chapter, we examine in more detail the role of moral judgement, and the emotion that often accompanies it, in everyday clinical work. In his book *Descartes' Error* (1994), neurologist Antonio Damasio makes a powerful case for the *essential* role that emotions play in human reasoning. To illustrate how emotion and reason interact, he tells a story about one of his patients. The patient had 'ventromedial prefrontal damage', damage to the frontal lobe of his brain, which left his rationality intact, but affected his emotional responses. Sometimes this emotionless reason worked to the patient's advantage. For example, on one occasion he arrived at Damasio's laboratory on a cold winter's day, when thick ice on the road led to extremely hazardous driving conditions. When Damasio inquired about the patient's journey, he was told it had been unremarkable and straightforward. The patient proceeded to detail for Damasio the proper procedures for driving on ice, describing how he had seen trucks and cars sliding and colliding and how he had been immediately behind a woman who had hit her brakes hard and skidded off the road and into a ditch. The patient recounted the incident dispassionately and described how he crossed the ice using his 'procedures'. He was emotionally unaffected both by any fear of the conditions and by the woman's misfortune. In these circumstances, the absence of affect was to his advantage, since he was able effortlessly to use 'pure' reason and steer his car across the ice.

However, the following day, Damasio, with the same patient, was attempting to agree a suitable date for their next appointment. He asked the patient to choose between two dates a few days apart:

> For the better part of a half-hour, the patient enumerated reasons for and against each of the two dates . . . Just as calmly as he had driven over the ice, and recounted that episode, he was now walking us through a tiresome cost–benefit analysis, an endless outlining and fruitless comparison of options and possible consequences . . . This behavior is a good example of the limits of pure reason.
>
> (Damasio 1994: 193)

In these circumstances, most of us would have become conscious of wasting the other's time. Crucially we would have *felt* embarrassed at making such a meal of a simple task and would simply have plumped for one day or the other. In these conditions, the emotions and the sensations that accompany them appear to be an essential accompaniment to reason.

It is rather the same with practice in health and welfare settings. If we are to undergo surgery, we may be thankful that a surgeon is not preoccupied with the perilous state of their marriage and the row they had this morning with their partner. However, if they discover some life-threatening condition inside our bodies we would hope that, when they come to tell us about it, they do not simply recite calculations about whether our expected quality of life warrants treatment, or adhere to some abstract ethical concept of autonomy and simply deliver the news and leave us alone with all the decision-making. We would want them to display feeling and care and help us to understand what we should expect. Emotional and moral judgements are therefore essential to 'humane' practice.

Yet moral judgements in professional work have had rather a bad press. Studies have tended to take a normative position and, when researchers find instances of professionals making moral judgements, they equate them with injustice, unfairness and the patient's loss of dignity. Writers typically invoke ironic contrasts between this identity-stripping (Goffman 1961) and a romanticized practice in which the patient or client is no longer victim of professional maleficence, but is truly valued by the clinician for their intrinsic human worth. Clearly, some of the moral judgements professionals make – for example, about good patients and bad patients – do indeed make us feel uneasy. They may certainly sometimes be unfair, and it is right and proper that these be made explicit and debated. However, we want to argue here that the moral aspects of professional work are a good deal more complex than these 'patient as underdog' positions imply. First, we want to argue that these perspectives tend to ignore the impact and relevance of *positive* moral evaluations of patients or clients. Second, much professional work is intrinsically emotional and moral. As we saw in Extract 4.6, professional anecdotes and homilies are frequently moral tales that transmit notions of what consitutes 'good' and 'bad' practice. Third, there are some areas of practice where pure reason cannot provide answers, even if, like Damasio's patient, professionals were able to use it. For example, child care social work depends to a large extent on moral reasoning. Social workers' talk is littered with references to 'appropriateness' and 'inappropriateness' and to whether parenting is 'good enough' (Hall 1997). The recognition that moral judgements are inevitable does not, however, mean that they are infallible. They are an important part of the tacit dimension of practice and, as we argued in previous chapters, as such they need to be defamiliarized, so we may properly debate them.

We argue below that practical–moral judgements are important in two principal and overlapping ways:

1   The characterizations and classifications of patients and clients in many service settings are ineluctably moral.
2   Professionals themselves are moral actors, who make moral claims about themselves and about other professions and agencies.

Both of the above are affected by, and in turn affect, the organizational, cultural and institutional contexts in which professional work takes place.

Good patients/bad patients

In his study of the typifications of good patients and bad patients used by staff in accident and emergency (A&E) departments, Jeffrey (1979) notes how patients may be assigned to one of the categories 'good/interesting' or 'bad/ rubbish'. 'Good' patients are those who allow the casualty officers to practise their skills and specialist knowledge, or who stretch their professional abilities but ultimately lead to them performing heroic or life-saving interventions. These patients are contrasted in the talk of A&E staff with 'rubbish', consisting of 'drunks', 'overdoses', 'tramps' and 'nutcases'. Jeffrey notes that patients typified as 'rubbish' break the following rules:

1   Patients should be responsible neither for their illness nor for their recovery. Medical staff can be held responsible provided they are able to treat the illness. 'Drunks' and 'overdoses' break this rule, as do people presenting with 'trivia' who could reasonably be expected

to manage their own illness and who deprive casualty staff of a proper role.

2   Patients should be restricted in their ability to carry on as usual. If they are not, they risk classification as 'trivia'.

3   Patients should see their illness or injury as an undesirable state. Obvious transgressors are overdoses and tramps: the former because they inflict the illness on themselves and the latter because they exploit the benefits of being a patient.

4   Patients should be cooperative in trying to get well. Again, overdoses clearly offend this rule, particularly if they repeat the attempt. 'Recidivists' brought in because of fighting or drunkenness also break this rule (adapted from Jeffrey 1979: 99–103).

While Jeffrey's work has been influential, it has been criticized and developed by other writers. For example, it has been suggested that Jeffrey pays insufficient attention to ordinary, unremarkable cases. This is important, since any area of practice will produce its own routine cases, which are processed straightforwardly with little explicit recourse to science, emotion *or* moral judgement.

Jeffrey's typifications have been further developed by Dingwall and Murray (1983), who use the concept of theoreticity derived from McHugh (1970) to add more complexity to the model. McHugh (1970) distinguishes between theoretic (an agent responsible for their own behaviour) and pre-theoretic (an agent who lacks the capacity to be responsible for their own behaviour) actors. These are moral categories that carry varying degrees of culpability for rule-breaking behaviour. Dingwall and Murray use this as a sensitizing concept to examine what happens to children in A&E departments. They note that children appear routinely to break all of Jeffrey's rules. They frequently injure themselves while undertaking some form of irresponsible act, such as leaping from a tree. The injuries are often trivial. Children often 'overreact' to their injuries by crying and screaming and can be exceedingly uncooperative. Yet children do not seem to receive moral censure. They are classified as pre-theoretic and are hence exempt from classification as 'bad patients'. Dingwall and Murray (1983: 140) produce the representation of moral judgements in the department shown in Table 5.1.

The term 'conventional' refers to situations where there is a choice to be

Table 5.1   Moral judgements in the A&E department

	Conventional	*Non-conventional*
Theoretic	Bad patients	Inappropriate patients
Pre-theoretic	Children	Naive patients

made; 'non-conventional' situations are those where there is no choice on offer. Once the model is complicated in this way, we can see that moral judgements do not flow straightforwardly from categories such as 'drunk', 'tramp' or 'overdose', but may be affected by the extent to which patients or clients are able to produce adequate moral accounts that may mitigate, explain or excuse their actions. So if a woman is admitted following an overdose that appears, on the face of it, to be a 'trivial' attention-seeking act, but during admission discloses that she has been subject to appalling domestic violence and psychological abuse, it is likely that she will escape any moral culpability. This means that we must pay attention to how moral adequacy gets 'done' and how it is judged in clinical work (Taylor and White 2000).

For example, the literature on parent–professional interaction in medical encounters provides compelling evidence of parents' sensibilities to the potential that they may be blamed by clinicians in some way. Parents must present their actions in the context of moral versions of responsible parenthood. For instance, in his work in a paediatric diabetic clinic, Silverman (1987) notes that moral evaluations of parenting depended on the extent to which parents were able to demonstrate that they managed and took responsibility for the child's condition, by monitoring blood sugar, administering or supervising insulin injections and providing a suitable diet. Decisions became more complex with older children, in relation to whom parents had to demonstrate that they were also encouraging autonomy. Stancombe's (2002) work on family therapy comes to a similar conclusion. He shows that the successful production of a moral account by a parent involves the use of one of the following sequences:

1   Parents present themselves as a 'good' parent who has done everything they can to ensure the welfare of their child and are continuing to act as a 'good' parent by seeking expert help for their child.
2   Parents may confess irresponsibility, admit to blame and seek absolution and so seek guidance, in the form of expert intervention, to ensure that they become 'better' parents.

We have more to say about the ascription of parental culpability in various settings in due course. However, clearly, the capacity to produce an adequate moral account is not evenly distributed and what serves as a satisfactory account is affected by institutional and organizational factors.

Moral judgements and organizational context

In her ethnographic study of nursing, Latimer (2000) examines the interface between acute and geriatric medicine. She notes that, in order to be a 'first class' patient, 'a patient must have a condition which may be considered *initially* as acute, but which has the potential for resolution so that he or she can be returned *in good time* to a category of patient which is dischargeable' (Latimer 2000: 23, original emphasis). These first-class patients are juxtaposed in nurses' talk with 'geriatrics', who are 'frail, old, gone off their legs a bit' (Latimer 2000: 23). Encounters with patients often entail the working up of distinctions between appropriateness and inappropriateness of older patients on the acute wards. Latimer describes one such case, Mrs Adamson, who was admitted with symptoms of breathlessness and chest pain, for which there were competing somatic (heart disease) and psychosomatic (anxiety) explanations. Discussions between nursing and medical staff focused on whether Mrs Adamson was 'really ill'. This distinction had particular moral consequences for Mrs Adamson.

> **Extract 5.1a**
> Throughout Mrs Adamson's stay the nurses kept in play the ambiguity over the cause of her troubles. At first, the nurses were very kind to her when she was distressed and having an attack of breathlessness and chest pain. But their ambivalence to her became more overt as Mrs Adamson's medical condition began to stabilize. The stability of Mrs Adamson's condition was constructed by the nurses' readings of Mrs Adamson's body, which returned to normal even though Mrs Adamson's troubles remained unresolved.
>
> (Latimer 2000: 61)

This led to the reclassification of Mrs Adamson's symptoms as psychosomatic, which caused a marked change in the nurses' behaviour towards her, with them becoming increasingly irritated by the time she demanded of them. This feeling was transmitted to Mrs Adamson in exchanges like the following:

> **Extract 5.1b**
> Mrs Adamson: I'm sorry, dear.
> Sister: Take nice deep breaths, none of these silly little pants. [Sister's voice has an edge to it, authoritarian, irritated.] No! Slowly, slow down – right [her voice begins to soften]. That's better, good.
>
> (Latimer 2000: 63)

Latimer is at pains to point out that this apparently hard and rather inhumane response is not in fact a reflection of heartlessness or lack of care, but a function of an organizational context, where ensuring an adequate flow of acute beds is a vital professional and moral imperative in itself. There is a complex relationship between the nurses' backstage contextualizing and reconfiguring work in relation to social aspects of patients' lives and the business of diagnosis itself. Thus, nurses' recasting of cases like Mrs Adamson's contributes to the flow of beds, essential in today's acute settings where success is measured by numbers of 'consultant episodes'.

Latimer stresses how bracketing the social aspects of a person's identity was crucial to ensuring flow through acute beds. Once 'socialized' a person's discharge became problematic. The distinction between medical and social is important in other settings, with each carrying varying moral connotations according to the context. If we go back to Jeffrey's work in A&E, he does not give a great deal of detail about the different narrative practices associated with cases, but he makes a very important observation: 'The features of good patients that are attended to [in professionals' talk] are medical in character, whereas rubbish is described in predominantly social terms' (Jeffrey 1979: 104). Thus, in a similar way to acute medicine, in A&E settings 'social' cases carry negative moral weight – they are seen as inappropriate.

Just as social cases are variously valued, so is attendance by clinicians to social matters. For example, in her study of life and death decisions in a neonatal unit, Anspach (1987) notes that physicians tended to rely on a combination of technological and perceptual cues:

> **Extract 5.2**
> Well, you really get dramatic kinds of information, I mean the baby's blood gases can improve or deteriorate markedly. I think that you can tell best in the nursery by your clinical exam unless something really gross supervenes, like congestive heart failure, and even more by how his laboratory parameters are doing . . . is this child gaining weight, are they having apneoic spells (episodes in which the infant stops breathing), you know, do his electrolytes, does his CBC (complete blood count), do his gases look good.
>
> (Anspach 1987: 220)

In contrast, the nurses tended to be among the first to raise questions about whether treatment should continue, warranting their claims using interactive or social cues such as the infant's responsiveness, eye contact and so forth which were not treated as reliable by the physicians. Anspach speculates that nurses' 'Continuous contact has its shadow side, permitting emotions (including negative ones) to develop, which may compromise the quality of an infant's care' (Anspach 1987: 227).

However, Anspach has little to say about *positive* emotional evaluations by the nurses and their possible contribution to decision-making, and neither does she engage with the moral status accorded to childhood and infancy in our culture. It is noteworthy that negative moral evaluations of older people appear to affect diagnosis and care, while those of infants do not. We have referred to Dingwall and Murray's observation that children appear to be a category exempt from classification as bad patients. There are particular moral domains relating to parenthood and childhood that are alluded to by such an observation. The observations in the following section are based on White's ethnographic study of paediatrics and child psychiatry and are developed further in Chapter 6 and in White (2002).

Moral judgements and child health: invoking parental love

Clinicians in child health settings routinely make distinctions between medical and (psycho)social cases. In this respect, paediatrics is similar to geriatrics, where, as we have noted, Latimer (2000) has shown how patients are constituted through professional talk as 'medical' or 'social'. Whereas in geriatrics the 'bringing off' of a social categorization is likely to result in patients being seen as inappropriate, or as 'bed-blockers', in child health services, particularly multidisciplinary ones, the classification 'psychosocial' still carries service entitlements, but of a different nature to 'medical' cases. We have given an example in Chapter 3 (Extract 3.1) of the very depersonalized way in which medical cases get told. Psychosocial cases differ markedly, as we can see in the extract below:

> **Extract 5.3**
> Michael Eaton is a five-year-old boy who was referred for behaviour problems, and when they came, Mrs Eaton has been very depressed for five years, she's had occasional admission to [psychiatric hospital], she's had cognitive therapy at [psychiatric hospital], she's had psychotherapy and counselling there as well that they'd organised. She's been on medication. Various different types and as I've said she's had inpatient admissions. Both Mr and Mrs Eaton say that Michael actually probably behaves much like any other five-year-old and that he doesn't have any problems, school aren't worried, they don't think he's got any problems, but Mrs Eaton can't stand him and that's the problem. She's very depressed, she can't bear him, she gets absolutely no pleasure out of his company whatsoever, ehm she you know to the point where she's actually got a two-year-old as well. She's completely bonded with the two-year-old and feels very warm towards him and deals with his misbehaviour perfectly appropriately but can't, when you see the two of them in a room when her eyes are on Michael she's all kind of gritting her teeth and by him and yet when she looks at Bradley, the younger one, she kind of softens and smiling and indulgent and ehm and she's broken hearted about this, but she can't stand her own son. Ehm we talked a lot about, I mean she's so depressed that, you know, her sort of negativity colours everything.

This is typical of the narrative practices in psychosocial cases. The emphasis is on the child's significant others, and together with assigning the mother to the membership category 'psychiatric patient', this establishes her responsibility for the problems. Anita Pomerantz (1978) shows how speakers use 'unhappy incident' reporting to accomplish blamings in talk. There are numerous such examples in this extract. The standardized relational pair (SRP) (see Chapter 3 and Glossary) mother–son is used to signal departure from category bound expectations and obligations (mothers love sons) and from category bound rights (sons are loved by mothers). In psychosocial cases this pairing often takes the place of the SRP doctor–patient, which situates the patient as worthy and the doctor as obliged to offer help for medical troubles. **Extreme case formulations** (Pomerantz 1986), which invoke the maximal or minimal attributes of a person or event, are powerful devices for referencing blame (or creditworthiness) in talk. These devices are common in psychosocial tellings (e.g. she *can't bear* him, she gets *absolutely* no pleasure out of his company *whatsoever'* 'irritated *beyond belief*', 'she's broken hearted about this, but she *can't stand* her own son'), and further facilitate the characterization of the parent both as failing and as deviant.

The account is also designed to convey intractability: 'Mrs Eaton has been very depressed for five years, she's had occasional admission to [psychiatric hospital], she's had cognitive therapy at [psychiatric hospital], she's had psychotherapy and counselling there as well that they'd organised. She's been on medication.' This is important in psychosocial cases, where there are few potent technologies for rapid relief. So invoking the list of 'tried and failed' here functions as a kind of prospective self-exoneration and 'expectation management' device for the clinician who is speaking. It helps to preserve her moral character. This is what Goffman (1959) calls impression management and it is a feature of professional work we consider in due course.

While many cases, like the one above, are already packaged (by the referrer) on referral to the services as 'psychosocial', this is not always so. Problems referred as 'medical' issues may, over time, become redefined (or socialized) into a psychosocial reading. In these cases, the paediatrician has powerful definitional privilege to adjudicate on whether it is the inside or outside of the child's body that is causing the trouble and judgements about parents are a crucial part of this process. We provide an extended example of this kind of case in Chapter 6.

White's study confirms and develops some previous findings. For example, it confirms Dingwall and Murray's (1983) assertion, which we discussed earlier, that children are a category exempt from classification as bad patients. While sometimes children or young people may be described as difficult, sensitive, challenging or damaged, this is attributed to their medical condition (e.g. they have autism), to their parents' or carers' (mis)management or to some other aspect of their biography. This includes those children and young people whose behaviour breaches moral codes – for example, those who self-harm, or engage in behaviour dangerous to others – and those whose chronological age places them very close to adulthood. However, Dingwall and Murray found that, in the A&E setting, moral judgement did not routinely pass to parents. This study confirms Strong's (1979) earlier findings that, in the more holistic domain of paediatrics, normative judgements about parents are a routine feature of the work.

There are two analytically separable but overlapping broad moral categories to which parents may be assigned. They may be classified as good/bad parents and/or as good/bad patients (although in reality they are patients by proxy only). A person may be deemed a 'bad parent' because they are believed to have wilfully neglected or deliberately abused their child, have put their own needs first or have acted in an evasive and deceitful way. These parents are in the theoretic category and almost always simultaneously defined as both bad patients and bad parents. However, as Strong (1979) also noted, references to parents' intellectual limitations are common in paediatrics. Parents may be described as 'not very bright', hopeless or helpless. Parents so described may have mental health problems or learning disabilities. While they may be seen as bad, or less than adequate, parents, providing they are help-seeking and help-accepting they may not be categorized as bad patients. That is, they are assigned to a pre-theoretic category (see above) and not held *morally* culpable for their poor parenting, even when they are dealt with in the formal child protection system. So while they are bad parents, they may still be 'good patients', who are grateful and can be helped. However, once parents breech the category-bound expectations (of themselves as parents and as users of expert help) to accept or follow advice, or do not 'see the need to change', they become potentially classifiable as both bad parents and bad patients.

In making their judgements, clinicians routinely refer to their 'feelings' about the family, often developed and reinforced by storytelling. In the following extract, a paediatrician is briefing a registrar about a family (the Kings) before an outpatient clinic. The consultant and registrar together work up a particular version of the parents, summarized by the consultant as follows:

Extract 5.4a

Con: The Kings, *Molly*, maybe you can have a dose of the Kings, you know her don't you?

Reg: Oh yeah, is she still as irritable as ever?

Con: (0.9) (laughs) It's her parents. It's their first child after trying for many years and they don't know anything about babies (0.4) so (0.4) they can't interpret anything from a normal perspective. They can't understand that whilst she was quiet when she was first born and she's irritable now doesn't mean that she's got a major pathology. She's just –

Reg: – awake and taking on the world

Con: Awake and irritable and life is like that really –

Reg: – yeah

Con: Every tummy pain, there has to be a sort of, every time she cries it must be her tummy. Although we showed that Infacol had no effect, didn't make any difference on the unit at all, they're really into the Infacol. Then, they're into constipation because if she hasn't pooed for so many hours then she's constipated. That's the problem, but having said that, just to fill you in Sue [directed to researcher], she has got a chromosome abnormality, so she isn't a – she was very small and is abnormal and we haven't got a clue what her outcome is going to be. It's understandable that they're having difficulty sorting out what is to do with her and what is to do with normal and you suggest things and in the end they do their own thing erm and it is really quite, quite hard work. So, so you'll, you'll have good time with them [to registrar].

By invoking their expertise and describing particular instances of the parents misunderstanding or disregarding medical advice, the doctors appear to be constructing these parents as potentially blameworthy as both bad patients and bad parents. There are apparent references to the breaching of a number of rules. In particular, the parents are typified as repeatedly present-ing 'trivial' symptoms and failing to take adequate account of expert advice. In response to this, White made an ironic remark to the registrar: 'Lucky you'. This was rapidly followed by a repair of her erroneous reading of the situation.

Extract 5.4b
Con: No they're very grateful and they're not –
Reg: Oh yeah they're nice enough parents –
Con: They're lovely, but they just need a lot of reassurance.

These qualitative judgements are particularly interesting, as the parents are clearly being classified as troublesome patients, but while perhaps 'naive' they remain morally good parents. This contrasts sharply with the case we consider in Chapter 6. Clearly the reference to parents' gratitude is import-ant and in keeping with the findings of earlier work. However, the references to the baby's smile are also relevant and later, in conversation with White after the clinic, the consultant draws explicit contrasts with the Chapter 6 case:

Extract 5.4c

Con: At least they're (the King family) saying isn't she lovely, have you seen her smile, she's pulling that funny face again d' y' know

SW: Yeah mmmm

Con: They're like, 'do you think that's a little bit of chromosome 9', whereas the mother upstairs [on the ward] would be 'well that's [ ] Syndrome isn't it, I mean look at her she's got this that and the other', not isn't she lovely she's my daughter.

In clinical practice, judgements about 'appropriate affect' form part of a repertoire of rationalities upon which clinicians draw in making sense of cases. Thus moral judgements in this setting are *affective* judgements. They are warranted in informal talk principally by the clinician's 'feel' for the family. There are no algorithms to help clinicians decide about the quality of love, but without these categorizations, the work of the clinic would be difficult or impossible. These kinds of positive moral evaluations are ignored in much of the literature on clinical judgement, although as we have shown they are resolutely part of professional competence.

Privileging the child's voice: negotiating blame in interaction

There are some particular consequences of the relative moral positions assigned to childhood and parenthood in child welfare services. When people present to services there are frequently competing accounts of the troubles that have led to referral. Gubrium (1992), in his ethnomethodological ethnography of family therapy, identifies the contextual practices in which therapists routinely engage to name, sort and categorize their experience of sessions and to make judgements about families' differing accounts and their lived realities. He identifies three 'rules', or 'taken for granted' practices, that therapists follow to depict domestic 'reality':

1   Ignore the constitutive work that the talk performs in constructing domestic reality. That is, treat it as a feature of the home and as a mirror on domestic reality.
2   Identify those features of the home that have supposedly produced particular features of domestic life. This involves the production of causal accounts of why the troubles exist and how they should be solved.
3   Use practical judgement to identify some feature of the family/ individual behaviour in the clinic setting as an instance of some

institutionally based theory; for example, relative seating positions in session.

Stancombe's discourse-analytic study of family therapists' backstage sense-making practices suggests that Gubrium's three basic rules require some amendment. The second rule should be reformulated to read: *'privilege the children's voice*, both actual and imagined, in identifying features of home that have supposedly produced particular features of domestic life'. Stancombe's data also provide evidence of a 'new' rule: 'produce versions of the troubles in which children never deserve blame or moral censure'. Moreover there is a corollary to this rule: 'even if they seem culpable it is because parents have been, or continue to be, deficient in meeting their emotional needs'. In combination with privileging the child's voice, this new rule effectively means that therapist formulations of the family troubles attribute blame to parents. Hence Gubrium's second rule should perhaps be more accurately described thus: 'identify those features of the parents that have produced the troubled child'. This tendency has also been noted by White (1997b; 2002) in relation to child care social work (see also Lloyd 1992).

In the following sequence, we can see how this is accomplished in backstage discussions between family therapists, a consulting team and the family's social worker. The family under discussion is comprised of a mother, a father and their two daughters, Sally (14 years) and Rachel (12 years). The family have been referred for family therapy by social services. The referring social worker (Gillian) was invited to the first session with the family and is active in discussion of the family troubles. The parents are concerned that their daughters are spending long periods away from home, sometimes overnight, without permission. They often stay with another family who live nearby. This family is 'well known' to social services. The parents have reached the point where they feel that all their efforts to limit their daughters' contact with the other family have failed. These efforts often end in serious confrontation and argument, and sometimes escalate to physical violence. The girls deny that they are at risk and resent their parents' attempts to restrict their movements. Thus far, attempts at conciliation between the parents and their children have failed. In the analysis below we concentrate on *how* the professionals construct moral identities for the family members, but this process relates to the question of *why* they do so; that is, the cultural moral value placed on childhood and the preciousness, passivity, vulnerability and corruptability of children.

Extract 5.5
1 Th: ((to social worker)) Do they (.) these girls show any (.) *stress* at
2   what's happening? Because they don't [in there
3 Cons1: [show it in there

4   SW: Certainly Rachel doesn't. Sally's not distressed. I think she's fed
5   up with the way things are going and really if only her mum and
6   dad let her do what she wants (.) life would be OK
7   Cons1: So she gets stressed by the arguments
8   SW: Yeah
9   Th: Though she's still not distressed by (.) for instance the breakdown
10   in relationships. I mean her mother said disintegration didn't
11   she? Such a strong word
12   Cons1: She said (.) psychological when she started (1.0) yeah =
13   Th: = No right towards the end =
14   Cons1: = Oh towards the end =
15   Th: = She said something about the family disintegrating. Something
16   about those different possibilities to prevent the disintegration
17   Cons1: And at the beginning she said I'm feeling desperate. That's
18   how she described her own feelings about what was happening.
19   You don't get any sense of that from the girls (.) at all =
20   Th: = Or from him actually. She's the one who communicates that
21   things are really awful. And probably if you were to meet the
22   father and daughters without her, you wouldn't get that sense at
23   all really. So I would guess that she is fairly kind of (.) isolated in
24   terms of the extent to which she feels this (2.0). But I guess that
25   these girls are so attracted by the excitement (.) stimulate – I don't
26   know how to describe it. Exciting. You know
27   Cons3: Den of iniquity =
28   Th: = Well yes
29   SW: That's what it is
30   Cons3: It is?
31   SW: Oh yeah. Certainly. The other people she mentioned are also
32   well known by social services. And I would have a lot of concerns
33   if they were my children with them (1.0) definitely (1.5) and
34   probably the drugs and the underage sex is quite a real issue
35   Th: But they're not able to even to register (.) that are they?
36   SW: Absolutely not. No. They were like (.) what's the problem (.) you
37   know. They're a great family. I really like them. And they listen to
38   me. So that's where they came in initially. Now I just think they
39   are looking certainly towards just to try and (1.0) rescue some
40   (1.5) part of the family really. Which we don't do that
41   Th: But it may be (.) like what they were saying (.) about being listened
42   to (.) I mean that may be a kind of crucial thing. I mean I don't
43   know. Maybe its gone too far past that and they've found this fam-
44   ily and they've taken everything that goes with it. Because some-
45   body's sat down and listened to them. If that's – 'cos that's what
46   they presented first of all didn't they? Not we can sit up all night =

47 Cons3: = We can talk to them =
48 Th: = We can talk to them. You know (1.5) all of them. The young
49   people and the adults can talk together and their friends eat
50   round there and (tails off)
51 Cons1: I suppose it's interesting that they are actually here, isn't it?
52   They could have voted with their feet. They do that regularly
53 Th: Well yes
54 SW: I mean the interesting thing was [mother] had agreed to tell the
55   girls about family therapy ehm but she hadn't done. That – and
56   then Sally of course came to see me and I'd been under the assump-
57   tion that she'd mentioned it and that was how I came to tell Sally.
58 Th: So I don't – yes. So. It would be interesting to find out (.) I mean
59   would it. What was it that prevented her from saying
60 SW: Mm . . . she didn't actually tell the girls that she contacted social
61   services at the beginning either. And hadn't thought that
62   through. 'Cos obviously I said (.) ehm (.) there is no way that I can
63   contact the girls directly if they're not even aware of who I am or
64   what I am doing (1.5) She says oh yes of course. So she then had
65   to raise that as an issue with the girls and check with them that
66   they actually wanted to see somebody as well.
67   (3.0)
68 Cons2: Some weird things got talked about for the first time in that
69   session, didn't they. With the girls actually bringing up trust.
70   Whether they can trust them
71 Cons3: Yeah. They're probably thinking what are their mum and dad
72   concocting =
73 Cons2: = Yeah =
74 Cons3: = all these plans without even ever discussing =

The extract opens with the therapist posing a question to the girls' social worker. This can be heard as a search for corroboration of one of her observations, namely that the girls do not appear to be overtly distressed by the troubles. The social worker is unequivocal in her response (line 4): 'Certainly Rachel doesn't'. However, she is more qualified regarding Sally ('I think she's fed up') and warrants this by invoking Sally's version of the troubles; the parents' 'unreasonable behaviour' is the problem.

Cons1 and the social worker then suggest that Sally gets 'stressed by the arguments' (line 7); the therapist moves to contrast Sally's apparent lack of 'distress' with her mother's version. However, the mother's actual use of language is selectively recalled and evaluated: 'her mother said disintegration didn't she. Such a strong word.' It is then contrasted with other versions in the family (line 17): 'at the beginning she said I'm feeling desperate . . . you don't get any sense of that from the girls (.) at all'. The therapist completes her turn with an implicit moral assessment of the girls' behaviour, the parents and the other family. The girls are said to be attracted to the other family by the 'excitement' and stimulation. At this point, Cons3 interjects (line 27) with an evaluation of M family household as 'a den of iniquity'. This implies that the parents' version, depicting the other family as morally inadequate, may be more credible and accurate than the version that the girls have supplied. The therapist's response (line 35) is somewhat ambiguous, in that it is not very clear as to whom the impersonal pronoun 'they' refers. If 'they' refers to the girls, it can be heard as the therapist reminding the social worker that the moral risk is not accepted by the girls in their version of the troubles. The social worker's response (line 36) suggests that this is how she heard it, and she proceeds to rehearse Rachel and Sally's version.

The therapist's next slot suggests that she hears the social worker's last turn as questioning the truthfulness of the girls' version. Between lines 41 and 46 she works up a version that constructs the girls' story of the M family as more factual and credible and also implies that the parents are guilty of neglecting their daughters' emotional needs. She begins with 'what they were saying about being listened to I mean that may be a kind of crucial thing'. In effect, the therapist suggests that the girls actively had to search for an alternative family to meet emotional needs neglected by their parents (line 43: 'Maybe its gone too far past that and they've found this family and they've taken everything that goes with it. Because somebody's sat down and listened to them.').

This is a quite explicit blaming of the parents, which is reinforced over the next few turns, where the social worker and the therapist together produce a story of poor communication between the parents and their daughters. The sequence opens (line 54) with the social worker reporting an 'unhappy incident'. That is, Mrs A had failed to tell the girls about the family therapy appointment, despite agreeing to do so with the social worker. The mother's failure to tell her daughters about the appointment and its 'unhappy' consequences further works to attribute blame.

The social worker goes on to produce a sceptical account of mother's communication with the girls. Initially, she appears to tell a story of unwitting neglect (line 61: 'And hadn't thought that through'), of the mother's failure to let the girls know that she was going to contact social services. However, there is a hint of irony in the social worker's story, as she tells the team about the mother's reaction to the social worker's refusal to make contact with the girls without warning (line 64: 'She says oh yes of course. So she then had to raise that as an issue with the girls'). This implies that perhaps the mother was more wilful in her neglect, and hence more culpable.

After a pause in the conversation, the therapists continue to make references to poor communication in the family that further assign blame to the parents. For example, they speculate that the girls cannot 'trust' their parents ('Yeah. They're probably thinking what are their mum and dad concocting . . . all these plans without even ever discussing'). Thus, Cons2 and Cons3 complete the blaming that was set up by the social worker's initial reporting of an unhappy incident. This accomplishes a moral evaluation of the parents, characterizing them as untrustworthy and dishonest, while at the same time privileging the girls' version of the troubles. This is despite of the fact that the parents have attempted to present themselves as appropriately concerned about their daughters' well-being and safety.

This extract has shown how a particular moral job gets done in interaction. We are not suggesting that it is wrong to privilege the child's voice. Instead we are suggesting that to do so is one significant component of the tacit dimension in child welfare work; so much so that the moral worth of practitioners is to an extent dependent on their ability to reproduce and display these valued cultural positions. The use of extracts of recorded talk can help to open up these dimensions for debate by practitioners themselves, so that they may properly evaluate whether they wish to use them on *this* occasion with *this* family (White 2001).

There are other moral aspects to getting clinical work done. In particular, professional work is rarely accomplished single-handedly and thus we are continually engaging in acts of persuasion to elicit responses from others. This work is generally invisible. It is only noticed when it is breached by someone who fails to follow appropriate rules of politeness (Brown and Levinson 1987) and to display respect for the other.

Producing moral selves: getting the job done

The work of Erving Goffman underscored the moral nature of interaction:

> [Face] may be defined as the positive social value a person effectively claims for himself by the line others assume he has taken during a particular contact. Face is an image of self delineated in terms of approved social attributes – albeit an image that others may share – as when a person makes a good showing for his profession or religion by making a good showing of himself.
>
> (Goffman 1967: 5)

Goffman reminds us that professional work is about more than technical competence. The dispersed nature of much clinical activity means that a great deal of time is spent on lubricating the social orders in which we work.

The following extract from White's fieldnotes is illustrative of the kinds of processes involved. The notes were taken immediately after observation of a paediatric outpatient clinic.

Extract 5.6

I arrived just after Greg (paediatrician) had taken in his first patient and I had to wait before joining him. When I entered the room, he told me he had just been seeing a 'little girl with juvenile arthritis who needs to have her knee injected'. He told me it was 'a nightmare to organize' because he had to arrange for the rheumatologist to go to theatre and inject the knee. The rheumatologist does not have any theatre time so he has to use the CPOD (pronounced ceepod) list (originating from the 'Confidential Inquiry into Perioperative Death'). I asked how the CPOD list was intended to reduce perioperative death and Greg replied 'by making sure surgeons don't operate at four in the morning'. Evidently the CPOD list is for emergency surgery but Greg told me 'it's not used for surgical emergencies'. He said, 'I'm always having to beg an anaesthetist to put her to sleep. Last time she came in starved at 2 p.m. and wasn't done until 5.30 p.m.'

Persuasion and flattery were used in getting the child on to the CPOD list. For example 'Hello, Dr Brown, I believe you are a very experienced anaesthetic registrar.' The explanation for the request was given as follows: 'Dr Ross doesn't have any theatre time. None of us has any theatre time. I'll put a cannula in her, because she has a needle phobia. Who do I book her with? The recovery staff? OK.'

Greg turned to me and said 'OK it looks like we can get her done.' However, there were still several calls to make which were fitted in between other patients. A telephone call was made to recovery staff – a good deal of repetition was required. Greg ended up shouting – as though to a person who was hard of hearing – not in an aggressive way. When he came off the phone he said 'One sandwich short of a picnic comes to mind – quite incredible.'

He told me how Clara will only allow him and nobody else to insert the cannula into her arm. It is clear that she is a special patient. He talked about how she needs to get used to other people, but when I said 'I think you're flattered really', he laughed and says absolutely.

The membership category 'little girl' carries certain entitlements of care and nurturance and moves the talk from the impersonal domain associated with the category 'patient'. We can see how Greg's clinical work is dispersed over time and space and the amount of flattery and switching of linguistic codes from esoteric to popular that is involved in getting this patient the theatre time she needs. Throughout this episode, Greg was explicitly displaying his care and concern for this patient, not as a dispassionate technician, but as a humane doctor. In conversation with the anaesthetist, he underscores his own unique role in the proceedings ('I'll put a cannula in her, because she has a needle phobia') and thus transparently references and owns the specialness of the patient and his relationship with her. The phrase 'one sandwich short of a picnic comes to mind – quite incredible' is an example of 'contrastive rhetoric', which is defined thus:

> An important feature of contrastive rhetoric . . . is the sometimes humorous but always dramatic definition of normality by reference to its opposite, deviance; and thus the demarcation (albeit a hazy one) of the outer limits of existing practice.
>
> (Hargreaves 1981: 312)

By using this device, Greg is able to produce his own competent moral self, juxtaposed with the incompetence, and by implication lack of appropriate care, of the recovery staff.

Thus, we have seen that moral work is intrinsic to getting clinical jobs done. Constituting our own moral character often depends on our drawing negative contrasts with that of others. Nowhere is this more evident than in multidisciplinary and multiagency work.

Contesting moral selves: blame and moral judgement in multidisciplinary work

> By casting occupation members as hero, atrocity stories maintain the intrinsic worth of the teller and, by implication, his colleague audience, acquiring an appropriate repertoire of such stories and being able to identify appropriate occasions for telling them are important parts of being recognised as a competent member of an occupation, or, more generally, any social group.
>
> (Dingwall 1977: 376)

Here, Dingwall is referring to the ways in which professionals tell elaborate stories about clients' and patients' antics or mishaps, and also about the incompetent response of some other professional or agency. In Dingwall's study of health visitors in training, he notes that the tutors often told stories about the incompetence or insensitivity of GPs, situating the health visitor as triumphant rescuer. For example:

Extract 5.7
Caroline: Why is the youngest child at risk?
Rosemary: He's retarded with a neuromuscular disorder
Pat: When was this found out?
Rosemary: The health visitor was worried quite early on, but the GP pooh-poohed it until after the developmental assessment.

In using the phrase 'pooh-poohed', the health visitor situates the GP as 'culpably wrong' and the herself as 'demonstrably right', thus reinforcing for the health visiting trainees the view that 'doctors should accord a more equal role to health visitors and not dismiss their opinions lightly' (Dingwall 1997: 381). This kind of storytelling is one way of accomplishing being a 'professional' and legitimating one's role alongside similar occupations. For example, in child care social work, pointing to the tardiness or inadequacy of other professions in the recognition of child abuse is a common 'atrocity story', which serves to reference social workers' 'monopoly expertise' and differentiate them from a range of child health professionals (White 1999; Taylor and White 2000). Once an individual has learnt through storytelling that a competent health visitor, therapist, psychiatrist, social worker or nurse thinks a certain way they are likely to reproduce these forms of thought as 'preferred' readings of cases.

In the extract below a child psychiatrist is discussing with a nurse manager some problematic cases that have been admitted via A&E to a paediatric ward over the weekend.

Extract 5.8
So we've got another problem brewing today which is Jessica Adams, who they mentioned on Saturday anyway. Ehm Jessica's again had a very bad weekend there's been a lot of violence at home. She's assaulted people, and I think she's been assaulted. She's come in with a black eye this morning in a very distressed state. Mum rang the Emergency Duty Social Work Team at the weekend and apparently got no support even though she'd been she'd had a foster placement until . . . last week. Ehm Mum rang me this morning saying I'm not prepared to have her home. Ehm because its just not safe its not safe for me and for the children because she's got quite young children. Ehm and it's just not working out. So I've asked her to ring the social work team, but her social worker's not in today so I said she needs to speak to the team leader and that we all do that as well as I wouldn't be at all surprised if they say that

they haven't got anything for her tonight and then she'll have to either go home or that we as a health service will have to provide something for her. I'll ask the paediatricians to look at her if she's been assaulted, and document its verging into child protection and both ways in terms of safety for Jessica and safety for the younger children.

And that's another one another grey case really that falls between us and social services. So there are I mean this whole issue of social services and our working relationship continues to be a problem . . . She doesn't need medication it doesn't make any difference when she's on medication. She was on . . . medication last time it made no difference . . . I said well you know if I came in, I wouldn't be doing anything. She shouldn't be on the ward. She should be you know in social services care. So it became a sort of psychiatric issue when it wasn't really a psychiatric or paediatric issue at all in the first place. Ehm but it does ehm it does cause a lot of problems really because I guess as psychiatrist I did my best to facilitate getting the [local area] psychiatrist to put pressure on social services to ehm to move things on really which I did do. I mean apparently at eight in the morning she didn't have a secure care place but by eleven she did. So you know there was movement.

This case involving a young woman with social problems, who is also showing a high degree of emotional distress, is situated at the interface between health and social care. These cases consume a disproportionate amount of clinical time, sometimes precipitate 'boundary disputes' between disciplines and often involve complex negotiations at the interface with other child welfare agencies and with NHS 'purchasers'. In the extract, the psychiatrist marks this case as 'trouble' with his opening utterance, 'So we've got another problem brewing today'. He then goes on to reference the case as 'social' by narrating the weekend's 'unhappy incidents' (Pomerantz 1978). However, in this context, these devices work to inculpate social services and not Jessica's mother, who 'rang the Emergency Duty Social Work Team at the weekend and apparently got no support'. The health service is depicted as the last defence against social services' failure. The reference to child protection marks the case as clearly social services' concern and prospectively constructs that agency as culpably negligent. The psychiatrist goes on to refer to another case, which he had described in detail earlier in the conversation. This serves to reference that Jessica's case is not an isolated incident. The non-psychiatric nature of the case is underscored: 'She doesn't need medication it doesn't make any difference when she's on medication. She was on . . . medication last time it made no difference . . . I said well you know if I came in, I wouldn't be doing anything.' Yet the final sentence situates the psychiatrist and by implication the health services as triumphant rescuers who have made social services face up to their responsibilities: 'she didn't have a secure care place but by eleven she did. So you know there was movement.'

Of course, the social services' version of this was very different. In their talk, the failure of the psychiatric system to provide proper help to young people who 'obviously had mental health needs' was underscored, with other similar cases cited as evidence. In the social services' version, it was the foster and residential carers left to look after 'very disturbed' young people with 'no support' who became the last defence against psychiatric failure. Each of these versions has its own truth and also speaks volumes about the malleability of diagnostic categories. That is, cases are often characterized by ambiguity, yet achieving disposal relies on the ability of the professional either clearly to claim the case as their own or to reconstruct it as the proper business of another profession or another agency. Through claiming or disclaiming a case, moral aspects of professional identity are performed, transmitted and reproduced. Talk about cases thus helps to differentiate particular professional identities from those of allied occupations and inducts novices into aspects of the tacit dimension. Moreover, it is an important aspect of multidisciplinary and multiagency work neglected in the current policy and practice literature, much of which simply exhorts that professionals engage in more effective communication with each other.

Summary

In this chapter we have argued that:

- The moral dimensions of clinical work are an important and under-explored area.
- It is commonplace for commentaries on professional practice to take a normative and evaluative position on the place of moral judgement in health and welfare services, typically constructing it as the root of 'oppressive' practices.
- Clinical practice is in many ways ineluctably moral.
- This has both positive and negative consequences which are likely to be local and contingent.
- What appears to be an unethical and inhumane response, may, in the context of some other moral imperative, make perfect sense (for example, ensuring rapid flow of patients in acute beds).
- There has been insufficient attention to the place of positive moral evaluations in clinical work.

- When transcripts of talk and similar materials are looked at in detail, it becomes possible to render explicit taken-for-granted aspects of professional moral orders. In so doing, the so-called tacit dimension is opened up for scrutiny and debate by professionals themselves.
- Professionals are moral agents. The performance of a moral self is central to clinical competence.
- Case formulations are often a product, at least in part, of professional identities, which are in turn reinforced by moral tales in the form of atrocity stories.

6 Science, morality and case formulation in paediatrics
A case study

In the previous two chapters, we argued, first, that science in its clinical context is often a negotiated and contingent matter and, second, that moral work of various kinds is indispensable in many, if not all, areas of health and welfare practice. In this chapter, we consider an extended case example from White's study of paediatrics. Using ethnographic fieldnotes and transcripts of meetings about the case, we show how forensic 'scientific' activity and moral judgement both play their part in the case formulation and how a particular reading is warranted in interaction, using a range of rationalities, including scientific knowledge, clinical experience and moral judgement. Before presenting the case in detail, we should consider some of the specific challenges involved in case formulation in child health settings. We argued in Chapter 5 that the distinction between medical and (psycho)social cases is important in many settings and we should consider in a little more detail the specifics of this distinction in paediatric services.

The problematics of case formulation in paediatrics

In keeping with other medical settings, the ordinary work of children's services is oriented to establishing relations of cause and effect. However, in child health, the attribution of causation can be particularly complex. Clearly, many children present to services with symptoms that may be unproblematically categorized and treated according to the established nosologies of biomedicine. Paediatrics has its share of ordinary, unremarkable cases. However, many cases are not so straightforward. For example, often children present with a physical complaint for which there may be a biological, neurological, genetic and/or psychosocial explanation. The obvious examples are enuresis (wetting), encopresis (soiling), constipation, various forms of developmental delay, communication or behavioural disorders and psychological distress. In accomplishing diagnosis and establishing causation in such cases, the boundary between problems with a biological and those with a psychological or psychosocial aetiology is particularly important for clinicians and is under-scored in professional literature (e.g. Garralda 1996; Woodward *et al.* 1998). The diagnostic categories themselves frequently reflect the same preoccupa-tion. For example, 'failure to thrive' in young children is routinely subdivided into organic (intrinsic) and non-organic (psychosocial) varieties.

The decision about whether a problem is seen to be part of the child's biological make-up or a product of their environment clearly has a direct bearing on the management of a case. For example, the suspicion that poor weight gain is not the result of genetics or a metabolic disorder, but is an indication that the child is not being fed or is emotionally deprived may precipitate referral to psychologists, child psychiatrists and social workers, rather than admission to a paediatric bed. The terrain is further complicated by the classification of a range of psychological or emotional sequelae to physical illnesses (e.g. Garralda 1994), which can create problems in the attribution of cause and effect. For example, are a child's frequent hospital admissions the result of intrinsic diabetic instability, a consequence of the child's emotional adjustment or of poor parental supervision, or do all three apply (Silverman 1987)?

As a result of these complexities, the same case may sometimes be told in many different ways in different settings and over time. Often, formulations shift when a new professional becomes involved and sees things differently. The propensity to see a case as either medical or psychosocial does not divide neatly by occupational group. For example, during White's fieldwork, a difference of opinion occurred between a child psychiatrist and a paediatrician over the diagnosis and management of a child referred because he was having 'funny turns'. The child psychiatrist hypothesized that this was epilepsy and ordered an EEG (a medical reading). The paediatrician, on the other hand, whom we might commonsensically assume to be less inclined to see potentially medical problems in relational terms, argued that the child was hyperventilating in response to problems in his relationship with his mother (a psychosocial reading). The EEG did not show any abnormalities, which was again variously used as a warrant for the very different case formulations. The paediatrician used it as confirmation of the psychosocial formulation, where the psychiatrist simply invoked the fallibility of the EEG as a diagnostic tool in the identification of seizures, arguing for more tests and observations. There is thus a strong case for examining the argumentative strategies professionals use when they work up versions of cases.

We have seen in previous chapters the very different ways in which medical and psychosocial cases are told, with the former characterized by depersonalized accounts and the latter by more florid storytelling, with detailed characterizations of significant adults. However, the most complex rhetorical work takes place in relation to children who have an identified and named 'medical' problem, which is generally agreed to exist independently of any issues about parenting, but this medical problem is thought to be being exacerbated by parenting practices (for example, children with unstable diabetes whose parents are suspected of mismanaging diet). Professionals do not have a discrete name for these kinds of formulation. They are identified by medical diagnosis, with accompanying narratives about parents/carers, or references to 'possible child protection issues'. The formulations can, however, be distinguished by aspects of their telling; for the purposes of differentiation, we have called them 'not just medical' cases (see White 2002). These formulations involve particularly complex storytelling, since the presence of an 'intrinsic' disorder requires that any psychosocial component be explicitly justified in the talk. Narratives about these cases have the flavour of detective stories with anomalous physical findings, such as failure to gain weight, set alongside characterizations of carers. Cases may begin as 'medical' and evolve gradually to a 'not just medical' or psychosocial formulation through formal and informal case-talk between professionals.

The natural and the social: 'not just medical' cases

'Not just medical' cases are common in paediatrics and are frequently referred on to child and adolescent mental health (CAMHS) or social work services. They are the most analytically interesting since, once clinicians have agreed that there is something medically wrong with the child, this skews the ages and stages of expectable physical, emotional and social development as calibrated by developmental psychology (White 1998). This makes the boundaries between normality and abnormality more fluid and contestable. For example, if a child has cerebral palsy and has difficulty swallowing and chewing, it becomes expectable that her weight gain may be slow. This exists as an available explanation for low weight and, in the absence of sudden and dramatic weight loss, clinicians need not necessarily investigate further. Further investigation must thus be triggered by something and this is often a highly contestable and practically onerous process, relying substantially on moral judgements and techniques of persuasion.

Asking the questions and undertaking the work to shift a case from a medical to a 'not just medical' formulation (or failing to do so) is not without personal risk. Parents who have a sick or disabled child may reasonably be expected to receive professional sympathy and support. Therefore, clinicians who raise concerns about parenting may be accused of zealotry or unnecessary punitiveness, but those who fail to explore some social dimension to the problem may (retrospectively) risk charges of naivety or collusion with parents if the child comes to any harm. It is for this reason that accounts of 'not just medical' cases often begin as 'fragile stories'. That is, they are defensively designed (Silverman 1998: 93) – oriented to the need to persuade and to the possibility of challenge. With repeated retellings and a receptive audience, they can attain the quality of certainty.

As well as requiring artful and persuasive telling, these formulations often involve practical detective work, rigorous questioning of 'witnesses', cross-checking of parental accounts and an almost forensic attention to detail. The following extended example shows the rhetorical and practical work involved in bringing off a 'not just medical' reading of a medical case. It concerns a child, Sarah, who has a rare syndrome, the name of which has been omitted to protect her anonymity. The syndrome is associated with multiple abnormalities. Sarah has had frequent admissions to hospital for a variety of reasons and the consultant has noticed over time that, on her return home, she loses the weight she has gained in hospital.

The first extract is taken from ethnographic fieldnotes:

Extract 6.1

I spent the morning with David one of consultant paediatricians. He took me to the ward to show me a 'very interesting case'. The case was interesting he said because it involved a child, Sarah, with 'lots of medical problems' who had been seeing nine different specialist consultants in various regional hospitals. David said that they were all 'only interested in their little bit' (of Sarah's body) and did not look at the whole picture. The child, aged 20 months, among other things had undergone heart surgery, had diabetes, and a gastrostomy, which allows her to be fed directly into her stomach. David told me that he had noticed that when the child was admitted to hospital she gained weight but would lose it again on return home. He said he suspected it was a case of Munchausen syndrome by proxy. The formulation was that, although the child had health problems, these were being exacerbated by the mother's management and that the mother was in some sense inducing the weight loss, by sins of omission or commission. There were some well documented feeding problems, for example, Sarah pulls at her gastostomy tube while she is being fed, which means that the food goes all over her and not into her stomach. However, David voiced real concerns about the way Sarah's mother presents. He says he doesn't think the mother is taking the time to feed Sarah and that she is 'obsessed with Sarah's medical problems'. We went down to the ward and met Sarah, who was on the playroom floor with the nursery nurse. She was linked up to a feed via a long tube on a mobile drip stand and was playing with bricks. David told me that she is very flat when she comes in but we 'lighten her up' whilst she's in – meaning that she is understimulated at home and improves in hospital.

We moved down the ward to look at Sarah's chart. There were lots of different weights recorded, and as they had all been taken on different scales, calculations were being done to make them comparable. David said that in future Sarah should be weighed on the same scales. David told me he needed to get the files from the other nine consultants from whom he has 'taken over'. He said, 'I need to look back at the other weights on previous admissions to see if she lost weight. That's work I haven't done.'

A long discussion ensued between David, the nurses and registrar about feeding problems. They decided to increase flow to 145 mls per hour and that Sarah should eat in an high chair with some food to play with so that it was a 'more normal experience'. They discussed the gastrostomy tube and asserted that it an 'adult responsibility' to make sure she didn't pull it out. There was an exchange of stories about visits from Sarah's mother. The new feeding regimen was written in the notes.

(Fieldnotes 13 October 1999)

In this extract, we can see the beginnings of a definitive re-reading of Sarah's case. The consultant's account begins by marking the case as 'very interesting'. It rapidly becomes clear that he is not referring exclusively to its 'medically' interesting features. He invokes the holistic moral role of the paediatrician in a district general hospital and juxtaposes this with the regional specialists, who were concerned only with those aspects of Sarah's body that were relevant to their domain. This provides an explanation and justification for David's reformulation, since he must account for why he sees the case in such a different way when nine other consultants before him have had no such concerns.

David is on tricky moral terrain, since Sarah has a serious and potentially life-threatening condition and accusing her mother of any form of abuse could easily be read as inhumane and uncaring. However, parents may well be exposed to professional censure in such cases, simply because the complex medical needs problematize the definition of what constitutes 'coping'. David not only refers to the medical problems but also alludes to the possibility of emotional neglect. Thus Sarah's mother may be vulnerable to censure on the two grounds Strong (1979: 52) outlines below:

it may seem that any mother could be easily idealized so long as she was relatively competent ... But whatever the actual qualities of a mother, certain medical conditions posed a serious and sustained threat to the easy achievement of the ideal. Psychiatric [psychosocial] cases and those of mental or physical handicap were equally dangerous, if in different ways. Severe handicap was an immediate challenge to a mother's capacity to cope and might also, particularly in the long run, threaten the affection and care that was a child's due. In [psychosocial cases] the parents might be the actual cause of a child's condition and, since the mother was the child's normal manager she must, it followed bear a large part of the blame.

(Strong 1979: 52)

In Sarah's case, dealing with the gastrostomy and the problems with the child continually removing it become part of the picture of a parent who is 'not coping' to an unacceptable extent. However, while 'not coping' is potentially a sufficient explanation for both frequent hospitalizations and the pattern of weight gain, it is only part of the formulation. References to the mother's presentation and demeanour, coupled with the observation that Sarah is 'very flat when she comes in but we "lighten her up" whilst she's in', mark the mother not just as not coping but as culpably failing or neglectful. The formulation depends on David's attention to detail in noticing the pattern of weight gain, but also on moral evaluations of Sarah's mother and her affective responses to the child. David refers explicitly to the need to do more work on plotting the patterns of weight gain and weight loss using notes from the other consultants in the case. He also takes steps to ensure that his own data are forensically robust, by ensuring that henceforth Sarah is weighed on the same scales each time.

Some weeks later, following further investigation into the pattern of Sarah's weight loss, a professionals' meeting was convened in the parents' absence, to consider the need to invoke child protection procedures in respect of Sarah. The transcript of the meeting is some 19 pages long. These extracts have been chosen because they illustrate the major strategies of argumentation and the various warrants used for a potentially contestable case formulation. David begins a long turn by outlining some of the Sarah's medical problems, specifically directing much of the talk to Jenny, the social work team leader, reflecting the purpose of the meeting (whether or not to use formal child protection procedures). While there is only one speaker for much of this story, the talk is clearly oriented to the possibility of reply; that is, to the audience and to the contingencies of the situation as social and consequential.

Extract 6.2

Right, OK, if I just take you through my report, Sarah's 20 months old now and I've only known her since July. She has [ ] syndrome and if you look at page 3 of your pages, [ ] syndrome is the name given to a child with a collection of differences . . . Right so as part of Sarah's [ ] syndrome she has a heart problem that has actually required surgery but is now off medication for that, she had a problem with her stomach and needed surgery on that, she's got a mild kidney problem and requires antibiotics for that, she's got some deafness and she's got a problem with one of her eyes and she's relatively short, so there are a collection of medical issues . . . when I took her over she was under nine different consultants for various bits of her care. When I do a full report I'll expand on all of those, Jenny (social work team leader), but I think it would take a long time to go into them and I think it's better to stick to the salient features of it really. I first met her because she came in with problems with diabetes, that is not related to the [ ] syndrome and she's also got asthma.

In this first extract, despite reference to her age, Sarah is located in the category of patient and the account is depersonalized with list of her clinical features. It reads like a medical case, but the explicit direction of the talk to Jenny the social work team leader alludes to what is to come. The case must at some point become constructed as the proper business of the social services department. The consultant continues by listing the care Sarah needs as a result of these complex medical problems.

Extract 6.3
She requires a certain amount of medical intervention. She can't chew and swallow normally so her main nutrition is through a gastrostomy but she needs feed to be offered you know smooth, like rusks, stewed fruit to be offered at meal times, alongside finger food which sometimes she takes and pump feeds via her gastrostomy for her main meals and for snacks, and she's fed through this gastrostomy of a night, so she's on a fairly hefty regime. She has inhalers for her asthma and night-time antibiotics to prevent infection and she requires hearing aids for periods of time in the day.

Here the consultant references Sarah as in need of particular sorts of care. In the next part of this turn, he invokes the technologies of paediatric medicine, such as the centile charts on which children's growth and weight are plotted. His account uses the language of scientific/forensic neutrality and objectivity and is linguistically coded as fact/certainty.

Extract 6.4
Now if you just look at this overall growth chart first, which is page 4 of your charts, you can see that she was born a couple of months early with her weight being on lowest centile which is the first centile and that she fell away from it. Now initially she had bowel surgery so we could understand that her weight gain wouldn't be that good, she had heart surgery half way through the first year of life but there has been a marked deterioration. Well a deterioration at six months,

deterioration and a marked deterioration at about a year, then effectively after the three months or even four months, after the first year of life she really didn't put on significant weight. So, the bit between the two arrows that looks a muddle on the chart, if you turn over to the next page I've blown the centile up so that the line you can see going through the circles is the third centile. That's the one across the top, the weight's on the left axis and the dates across the bottom. The bits highlighted in pink refer to the hospital admissions, the first admission had the most dramatic weight gain, but she was ill at that time with diabetes so a considerable amount of that would have been because of that, so say 1 kilo of that or the first little rise would have been the fluid, but there does seem to be a pattern of rapid weight gain in hospital and a tendency to plateau or lose weight on going home. The distance from the third centile, we'd got her on the 6th August, we'd got her really approaching the third centile as near as she'd been to the third centile for a long time. If you look back she was back to where she was at three months of age and we've lost the distance from the third centile since. So . . . these weight gains are quite . . . I mean this is a 3 lb weight gain . . . I mean she was 8 kilos and had gone up to 8.8 which is getting on for 2 lb in weight and she's been in hospital a week. You must remember that some of the difficulties with the weight will depend on when she's being weighed in relation to her feeds because she does have a bolus of feed, so if it's after a bolus she will weigh more.

We can see referenced here the forensic work of the consultant, both in ensuring the child is weighed at the same time in relation to her feeds and in annotating and highlighting the various charts so that their salient features are recognizable to a mixed professional audience. Throughout this account, the consultant presents potential alternative readings of the periods of weight gain and weight loss, demonstrating that all things have been properly considered. Rather than casting doubt upon it, this 'hedging' works to reference the trustworthiness of the primary formulation.

This is followed by references to the social/emotional aspects of development, which leads to a summary of the formulation so far, invoking the legal concepts of 'avoidable impairment' and 'significant harm' imported directly from the Children Act 1989. This achieves the construction of the case as multiagency business and relies on the paediatrician's category entitlement to adjudicate on 'significant harm' in sick children.

Extract 6.5

Can I take you through the rest of the thing [report] and then we'll take questions because there are . . . also of concern the last three admissions have been associated with significant lethargy and Sarah appearing less motivated and interested in her environment and learning. We haven't, well maybe Anne (nurse) has more documentation, we'll come round to Anne in a bit, can't we really but her development seems to spurt on or her interest or her liveliness seems to improve in hospital and then when she comes in we're feeling that we're going back a step and we've got to work on getting her going again. Then I basically go on to say in view of these experiences with Sarah's weight our concern that Sarah could be doing significantly better and that her growth and development are being avoidably impaired, i.e. she's suffering significant harm. A significant, prolonged improvement in weight gain would also lead to an improvement in height and head circumference which would enable Sarah to consolidate her development.

This formulation is supported in the next extract by characterizations of Sarah's mother. This is a potentially contentious issue, as we noted above, since caring for a child with this range of complex medical needs may reasonably be expected to provoke professional sympathy. Here, the consultant invokes his status as eye witness: 'I have also observed the following.'

Extract 6.6
I have also observed the following. The mother concentrates on the medicalization of all Sarah's care. When she first presented she went on about all the nine consultants she was under, the number of medical problems that she had, that she was very difficult to manage that no one would be able to manage her medically and questioned us to how many children with [ ] syndrome I've managed and that they were totally unpredictable. She appears to have a very negative outlook for Sarah, she wasn't going to grow, she wasn't going to develop, she was going to go to a special school and her husband hadn't really taken any of this on board . . . Her mother has also said that if Sarah puts on weight it will put a strain on her heart and she will die of heart strain, I've reassured her that that's not true and if she doesn't put weight on she won't do lots of other things. She's convinced that there is more and more wrong with Sarah.

The account is linguistically coded as fact, not opinion: 'the mother concentrates on the medicalization of all Sarah's care'. To a lay reader this may seem a rather strange statement, since much of Sarah's care is self-evidently medical. However, this is the first stage of a process of argumentation designed to persuade the audience that this is indeed a case of Munchausen syndrome by proxy. Use of irony such as 'she went on about' and accounts of the mother's questions about the consultant's expertise serve to signal that this mother is a 'troublesome patient by proxy'.

David completes his turn by reporting the mother's 'admission' that she isn't feeding Sarah as she should during the day.

Extract 6.7

Cons: When asked about why she puts weight on in hospital but loses it at home she says that's because she's always ill at home and it's the illness that you can't find that is causing this problem. During the first admission she admitted she wasn't feeding her in the day like she should have been, she was missing most feeds but perhaps giving her a small amount at lunchtime. She said that she often smelt of ketones and smelt like pear drops which she had mentioned to numerous doctors and that's the smell you get when you're starved and that they haven't looked into it.

Team leader: Did she say why she wasn't feeding her?

Cons: Well, you see, you get up and you have to take the others to nursery so there isn't really time and then she goes to CDU [child development unit] so there's no time, and then she has this appointment and that appointment and then there's no time and then she's picking the children up from school and there's no time.

The consultant's second turn is heavy with irony and he continues by recounting all the efforts that have been put in place to assist. He uses the reported speech to reinforce the mother's culpability. She is constructed not just as 'not coping', but as 'not caring' (Hall and Slembrook 2002).

Extract 6.9

And I then said well let's rationalize the appointments because the main thing is that you have time to feed her and if she hadn't got her problems you would have to give her breakfast, you would have to give her – which might take quite a long time if she's a toddler, you'd have to give her a drink and a biscuit in the middle of the morning, you'd have to give her lunch and a drink and a biscuit in the afternoon, and you'd have to give her tea and you'd probably have to give her supper. 'I'd hadn't thought of it like that, I'd probably have just given her a rusk and sat her in the car' is what she actually said and I said what would you have done if she was hungry and she said 'given her a rusk while we drove to school', she also said, as I've said though this is an extremely brief report Jenny really.

In the following summary, David again quotes directly from the Children Act 1989: 'I'm concerned that his growth and development are being avoidably impaired'. This displays his expertise in child protection matters. He also makes explicit reference to the possibility that Sarah's mother is *deliberately* manipulating Sarah's weight.

Extract 6.10

Either by inadequate feeding, or by other manipulation. She's also said and I forgot to put this in the first bit, that she will pull the plug out of her gastrostomy and she'll find the feed has leaked into her nappy or into her cot, and I said well you need to stop her and if it's all come out you need to put it back in and feed her again. And there's one thing after another as to why this hasn't been in – so whether she's not feeding her, or whether it's coming out again. She has had diuretics, that's water tablets, in the past for treatment of her heart and the rate of weight loss and the rate of weight gain is so dramatic that I'm wondering if she's actually giving her diuretics, because there have been times when her weight has been relatively static at home and she has clearly wanted me to readmit her and I've said no, you have her another week, you've got to do it at home and the next week, you can bet your bottom dollar really that within a few days she'll be in and her weight will have fallen off.

The explicit suggestion that Sarah's mother may be 'actually giving her diuretics' is necessary rhetorical work in order to close down an alternative view of the case which has been gently alluded to by one of the participants in the meeting, a specialist health visitor, who observes:

I was just reading the bit about most children with [ ] syndrome are dead by the age of one year and she is still referring to that. That can have a tremendous effect on people, they may withdraw themselves believing they will protect themselves.

The suggestion that Sarah's mother may have some kind of depressive grief reaction to Sarah's prognosis would exculpate her from the 'not caring' version that David is trying to present and reassign her to the less morally problematic category 'not coping'.

The formulation of Munchausen syndrome by proxy also requires David to establish that Sarah's medical problems are not the cause of the weight problems and this involves a degree of minimization in response to a question from the social work team leader.

Extract 6.11

TL: What about her heart problem, has that been resolved?
Cons: She had two holes that she's had closed and she has a trivial leak

in one valve that is probably not of any consequence but it needs monitoring. Her kidney problems should be resolved by the age of five, she's got asthma which a lot of children have, she's got diabetes which is in remission now and may stay in remission for a number of years ... her main problem is the gastrostomy and the feeding and her coordination but then it's difficult to know how far that could be brought on with perseverance with offering appropriate food.

Here, the leak is defined as 'trivial', the kidney problems as 'resolved', the diabetes as 'in remission' and the asthma as something 'a lot of children have'. The main problem is feeding – recognizable to the audience as a normal trouble of childhood with which 'coping' parents may reasonably be expected to deal. Further character work completes the formulation.

Extract 6.12
I don't personally believe that the maternal instinct, or whatever, to have a child in the house of Sarah's age, not be able to feed her and not have any feelings of need to feed her. Most parents would not be able to tolerate that. They would be force feeding the child, they would be beside themselves with worry about her not eating and there's none of that. She could go through a day and she would have 50 mls which is less than 2 oz of feed in a whole day and she would not be anxious about her. And if someone is at that level of dysfunction for whatever reason, I mean I don't know if there are elements of, if you think of the Mary Eminson scale of illness perception you know from neglect to the frank Munchausen, I would see her as scoring fairly high. I'm not sure if she's in the neglect end, which is where a lot of the failure to thrives are, I think she's more the excess perception end, making a problem end. She's sort of creating situations if you like.

Here the voice of science (the Mary Eminson scale) and the category entitlement of the consultant to adjudicate on good enough parenting combine to produce a powerful case. Noteworthy also are the use of contrast structures (Smith, 1978), the first half of which set up an expectation of proper behaviour and the second a deviation from it. For example, 'Most parents would not be able to tolerate that. They would be force feeding the child, they would be beside themselves with worry about her not eating and there's none of that. She could go through a day and he would have 50 mls which is less than 2 oz of feed in a whole day and she would not be anxious about her.' These devices also reference deviation from category-bound obligation expectations of parenthood.

The paediatrician's turns are followed by detailed accounts given by nursing staff of the mother's behaviour on the ward and of Sarah's presentation on various admissions. There is some discussion about whether further work is necessary to gather more evidence, or whether the case should be taken into the formal child protection system. The team leader summarizes this discussion as follows:

Extract 6.13

TL: To use case conferencing positively, which is the way it should be used, you would go in and say this is the purpose of the case conference to bring everyone together, to get consent and plan. If you do it that way, you can use the case conference. If you intend to plan and then say go, we'll go to conference, it's usually like a punishment which it's not because it's there to provide support . . . But, in a way, the last meeting you had before they went home was a support package, in a way you know.

Cons: That's how I feel, I offered [local support service]. We reinforced the feeding. We reinforced the hearing aids and there's not really any evidence that any of that has been taken to fruition and OK it was a low-key planning meeting, but nevertheless the elements were there. The health visitor was there, the CDC staff were there, the hearing support teacher was there, Mandy [home care nurse] was there, [local support service] were involved. We bent over backwards to try and listen and sort things out for her.

TL: The other thing that the case conference will serve to ensure is that social work should undertake an assessment of the family situation which is what you need as well.

Cons: Well, I think that's what we need mostly, because . . . Sarah's mother, in my view, has major problems and I'm not really sure what the nature of these problems is, and how treatable those problems are and how much this is personality that won't change and how much this is a protective mechanism from the desperate situation that she thinks she's in.

In her first turn, the team leader is producing a moral warrant for taking the potentially controversial step of moving this case, involving a child with such serious medical issues, into a child protection arena. Throughout the account, the team leader and consultant are arguing the case together. The team leader's first utterance draws on her knowledge that, in order to justify taking a case to conference, it must be demonstrated that 'family support' has failed, or that the level of risk is too great to attempt such an activity. However, it is delivered not as a challenge to the consultant's reading, but as a ready-made rationale for taking the child protection route. The list of 'tried and failed' interventions given in response by the consultant reinforces the argument in favour of a child protection intervention. The allusion to the mitigatory potential of the mother's psychological problems is delivered ironically: 'and how much this is a protective mechanism from the desperate situation that she *thinks* she's in'.

The end of the meeting is devoted to planning the encounter with Sarah's parents and how the team leader may best be involved in this.

Extract 6.14

TL: I think that either myself or Kay [job-share team leader] can come in towards the end of the interview and meet the parents. I don't mind which it is, to do the whole interview, or half of it, or come in at the end, whatever you decide.

Cons: I'll see when they can come in. I would perhaps like to start it off myself and say, 'look I've been assessing the situation, I know we've found these bits, but this is the reality and clearly things are happening at home that aren't doing her as well as those that happen in hospital and that has to change.' Then, if you could be around to take on the planning bit and the idea of a support package, but through a case conference. I'll bring that up as well.

This was precisely the way the case was managed after the meeting, with the concerns presented to the parents and a case conference held shortly afterwards. There are clearly alternative ways in which this case may have been understood. For example, Sarah's medical needs could have remained the primary formulation, with the mother's reactions constructed as 'understandable in the circumstances'. This particular reading relies on strategies of argumentation and persuasion, considerable behind-the-scenes detailed forensic detective work on the part of the consultant and nurses, an audience with a shared professional understanding of 'significant harm' and the category entitlement of the consultant paediatrician to authorize the bracketing of Sarah's medical problems. The formulation depends not only on centile charts and scales, but on the working up of a convincing characterization of the mother and on the availability of the nosological category Munchausen syndrome by proxy. In the meeting, all these warrants are treated with equal evidential weight. In particular, the use of irony and moral reasoning signals the importance of the 'affective' judgements we discussed in Chapter 5. It will be instructive if we examine again how David accounted for his different reaction to another family:

Cons: At least they're (the King family) saying isn't she lovely, have you seen her smile, she's pulling that funny face again d' y' know

SW: Yeah mmmm

Cons: They're like, 'do you think that's a little bit of chromosome 9, whereas the mother upstairs [on the ward] would be 'well that's [ ] syndrome isn't it, I mean look at her she's got this that and the other', not isn't she lovely she's my daughter.

Summary

This chapter has shown how complex are the forms of reasoning used by clinicians in a paediatric service when they try to establish relations of causation. Shared understandings of patients and their troubles emerge out of interaction between professionals. By examining how clinicians tell cases, we can see how science, seasoned professional 'know-how' and moral judgement coexist as warrants for action. As we noted in Chapter 5, moral judgement in this context is usually 'affective' judgement, and is warranted in informal talk principally by invoking emotion: the clinician's 'feel' for the family or for the appropriateness and/or inappropriateness of parental 'affect'. So in Sarah's case, David's clinical scientific work was motivated largely by his affective judgement of Sarah's mother. Clearly the science also had to 'fit', but his principal warrant for undertaking the forensic work in the first place was Sarah's mother's emotional presentation, inconsistent stories and general 'oddness'. Of all the health and welfare occupations, medicine is the most conventionally scientific, yet as Strong (1979: 214) notes, 'far from being neutral scientists, doctors can appeal to the neutrality of "natural" science in order to conceal the systematic moral investigation and judgement in which they are engaged.'

The stories clinicians tell have clear material consequences for the various parties to the case. For the families in 'not just medical' cases there are a number of clear consequences. The amount of professional time, the number of professionals, the range of services involved and the amount of time spent on coordinating activity increases as the zones of relevance expand outside the child's body to include family and social relations. Once these zones are opened to professional scrutiny it is rare indeed for a case to revert to a purely medical formulation, as more information usually breeds continued concern. In these cases, the professional encounter with the family also shifts in focus and style, becoming more confrontational and interrogative, as clinicians address moral questions about the parents' capacity for change, or about the extent to which they have 'taken responsibility' for the problem, as we can see in the final extract above.

The consequences for families of 'not just medical' reading may be both positive and negative. For example, Sarah's name was subsequently placed on the register of children at risk and a formal child protection plan instigated. This sustained the high levels of service provision and no doubt kept Sarah safe. However, it also increased surveillance and censure and silenced a potential alternative reading of the case where Sarah's mother may have been constructed as a distressed or depressed parent who was struggling to care for her child and needed help, but was not herself morally culpable for the predicament. She could have been constructed as caring-but-not-coping (Hall and Slembrook 2002).

It is not the purpose of this chapter to adjudicate on the correctness of decision-making in relation to the case presented. Instead, we have sought to illustrate the complexity and ambiguity of many presenting problems in child health care. The protocols and procedures of scientific-bureaucratic rationality provide a poor fit with these ambiguities. In their clinical work with such cases, professionals carve certainty from uncertainty, not only by weighing and measuring or consulting guidelines or protocols, but by engaging in moral reasoning and artful rhetoric and persuasion. In working up causal accounts with other professionals, clinicians do not simply draw upon an external body of knowledge, but are literally *arguing* the case. If clinical judgement is this complex, we should not be squeamish about saying so. It is only by acknowledging the importance of moral judgement that we may engage appropriately with the practice implications. We consider the implications for professional education and practice in more detail in Chapter 8.

7 Managing multiple versions
Rhetoric and moral judgement in a family therapy case

Throughout this book, we have argued that the judgements clinicians must make are frequently influenced by emotional, historical, social and cultural factors. That is, judgements cannot be reduced entirely either to the neutral application of knowledge, as is presumed in technical and procedural models, or to individual cognitive processes, as is assumed in much of the psychological literature (see Chapter 1). Instead, judgement often depends on interactive processes between the clinician and patient or client and between the clinician and their colleagues. In Chapters 5 and 6, we underscored the importance of morality in professional decision-making. In this chapter, we explore this further by examining what happens when clinicians attempt to 'do' moral neutrality. In this context, family therapy provides an illuminating example, since it is explicitly wedded to an ethic of neutrality. The therapist is typically depicted as an expert in conversation who can move family members from particularly unhelpful and morally loaded positions to accountability-free ones in which positive change can more readily occur.

The pursuit of openness is typically seen to depend on the therapist maintaining a non-partisan position in relation to the versions of events presented by family members. In family therapy, the concept of neutrality was given theoretical prominence in the work of the highly influential Milan school (Boscolo *et al.* 1987), and, as a result of its critique (see, for example, Golann 1988; Frosh 1991; Goldner 1991; Epstein 1993), 'multipartiality', 'not knowing' and 'curiosity' have emerged as the canons of contemporary practice. For example, Epstein and Loos (1989: 416) maintain that therapists 'must develop a position that simultaneously respects all the views of all the participants'. Therapists, then, are meant to be, or at least to act as though they are, morally neutral. In this chapter we want to challenge this notion of neutrality as an ethic or trait internal to the therapist and to argue, in keeping with the theme of the book, that it is better seen as something far more interactive. In the context of television news interviewing, Clayman has noted:

interviewees, by virtue of their concrete participation in the encounter, necessarily contribute to the overall sense and appearance of interviewer conduct, suggesting that received notions of neutrality (for example as a trait that interviewers possess) may have to be reconsidered. The visibility of this journalistic 'trait' is in many respects a collaborative achievement.

(Clayman 1988: 475)

This point is echoed by Greatbatch and Dingwall in their work on divorce mediation: 'The ability of individuals to maintain a neutralistic stance in talk-in-interaction is dependent upon the co-operation of other participants' (Greatbatch and Dingwall 1999: 274).

The point these authors are making is that neutrality is something that requires collaborative work. Possessing a motive of neutrality is no guarantee that one's utterances will be heard or treated as neutral. There is plenty of room for misunderstanding and suspicion. By subjecting therapists' and families' talk to detailed analysis, it is possible to show that neutrality is indeed an interactional accomplishment.

The moral context of family work

[The] not-knowing position entails a general attitude or stance in which the therapist's actions communicate an abundant, genuine curiosity. That is, the therapist's actions and attitudes express a need to know more about what has been said rather than convey pre-conceived opinions and expectations about the client, the problem or what must be changed . . . This allows clients room for conversational movement and space, since they no longer have to promote, protect, or convince the therapist of their view.

(Anderson and Goolishian 1992: 29–30)

This is a familiar and appealing argument, articulated from the 'neutrality as ethic' position. However, we shall go on to show that it ignores the morally laden nature of work with families and also the social meanings ascribed to therapists failing to take a position. Anderson and Goolishian argue that the adoption of a not-knowing position frees clients from the imperative to persuade the therapist to take their side. Yet, when families come to therapy, their members are usually engaged in some form of mutual recrimination. If they are vocal, the first task of individual members in therapy is often to recruit the therapist into their own particular reading of events, as Buttny notes:

> The discourse of relational problems often takes the form of the teller describing him/herself as reacting to the unjustifiable actions of his or her spouse – 'You (actively) did something to (passive) me and I (having no choice) had to respond as I did' (Lannamann, 1989).
>
> (Buttny 1993: 66).

Previous discourse analytic work has shown that family members make use of sophisticated linguistic strategies in these attempts to persuade. For example, they often anticipate the charge of bias or partisanship and use strategies to defend themselves against such accusations (for example, Cuff 1993). Having undertaken this rhetorical work, they are likely to be very vigilant in their attempts to deduce whether the therapist has 'bought' their version. This makes the imperative to display neutrality somewhat precarious for the therapist, as being non-judgemental or silent on a topic can easily be read as dismissiveness, failure to understand or evidence that they are unconvinced by this particular family member's version.

In short, families come to therapy as members of society, and as such they use the range of interpretive techniques that we all mobilize routinely in making judgements about the supportiveness, trustworthiness and authenticity of others we meet in everyday life. This interpretive template is ready-made before therapy and may be resistant to modification whatever the skill of the therapist. In short, families may simply fail to 'get it' when therapists do neutrality and 'not knowing'. So, in the sea of versions, the therapist runs the risk of being heard to side with one member's version over another; and thus to join, at least implicitly, in the attribution of blame. Or they may alternatively leave members feeling that their versions were unconvincing, or have been ignored or misunderstood.

This chapter concentrates on how therapists manage these multiple versions of the troubles that routinely arise in therapy with families. It concentrates on one case, the D family. The therapist is working with the mother and her two teenage children, Chloe and Steven. The father is not living with the family and is not part of the session. The mother's account of the troubles casts her as 'victim' of the unreasonable behaviour of both her children. In contrast, Chloe argues that she is the main victim of her brother's outrageous behaviour. She also blames her mother for failing to protect her from her brother's aggressive behaviour. Steven says very little in defence against these allegations. We begin the analysis by looking at how, in this atmosphere of mutual recrimination, the therapist attempts to convey neutrality in this session. We then examine how the family members' versions are discussed and reformulated during a mid-session consultation with colleagues who have been observing the therapist and family behind a screen, and finally how the therapist manages the feedback to the family. We show how doing neutrality appears to have a number of paradoxical effects, which suggest that moral judgement simply cannot be avoided. The case example has been chosen for its typicality, and is drawn from a substantial corpus of data. However, see Stancombe (2002) for a full discussion of the range of strategies used by families and therapists to negotiate moral matters.

Doing neutrality in talk with families: the first paradox

There are two principal strategies that therapists use to negotiate the morally laden stories family members tell. The first of these is simply to ignore the family member's account and change the subject, and the second is through the production of preliminary (re)formulations of the versions offered.

Changing the subject: the risk of not being heard?

Extract 7.1

Ch: I s'pose I'd agree with him they're better. 'Cos he doesn't (.) hit me. (1.5) It's just (.) he's start – (.) he always has gone in my room. But (.) he goes in (.) he used to know where I hid my purse. He's broken my stereo 'cos he took it on his paper round. And that was something someone bought me. Ehm. He'll just go in and take batteries out of things so he can use things. I came home last weekend and all my drawers were open. And I'd shut my door before I went out. And I knew he'd been in. He went in. And he roots through everything so he can find things. (2.0) And he just thinks there's nothing wrong with it. (2.0) To be rooting through all my private things 'cos now I've got my own room. (2.0)

Th: Did you used to share then?

In this case, the therapist's change of subject could have a number of functions. It may have been utilized to manage the overt blaming of Steven by his sister, which was inviting the therapist to sympathize with Chloe and express moral censure of Steven; thus challenging the therapist's neutrality. The change of subject may also have been used to save Steven's face, and prevent further overt blaming of Steven, with the likelihood that he would not want to return for further meetings. However, while the therapist's manipulation of the conversation achieved closure on the blaming in the session, this form of blame management runs the risk of leaving the member who is telling the story feeling unheard.

Moreover, it increases the likelihood that the teller will feel the need to reiterate their story, or versions of it, later in the session. Indeed, in the following extract, taken from later in the session, Chloe can be heard telling almost exactly the same story of her brother's maltreatment of her as she narrated previously. This is ushered in by the mother's account of her son's stealing habits.

Extract 7.2

Th: Is, is that normal (.) that Steven's been able to say (.) yes I did that and
    [(   )]

Mo: [The trouble] is it happens so often that (.) I, I mean her polos dis-
    appeared you know but (1.5) short of having closed circuit TV in his
    bedroom I, I mean her bedroom. (1.0) But you I mean things dis-
    appear and you've got a pretty good idea where they are. I hate it
    when I can't trust anybody. (2.0). That really irritates me. But I don't
    think it's him I think it, it's you know I thought it was just *him* (.) and
    you feel guilty (.) b-but other people's kids at work have done it so
    it isn't just (1.0) it isn't. (2.0)

Ch: But he roots through my drawers to find my things. I hide things in
    different places but every time he's found it. And then he finds the
    new hiding place. Now I can't use my stereo at all 'cos that doesn't
    work. Somebody bought me that for my birthday. (2.0) He stole
    sweets off me and money off me. And I know I shut my door
    on Saturday night. All the doors were closed. And I have this thing
    where I kept my polos which he knew about. When I came back
    the drawers were open. He hadn't shut them properly. My door was
    open. I knew my Mum hadn't been in. So the door should have been
    shut still. (4.0)

Th: What is the arrangement w-with pocket money and stuff 'cos

The mother's utterance conveys that she is not culpable for Steven's stealing: 'I thought it was just him and you feel guilty but other people's kids at work have done it.' She also emphasizes the great efforts she has made to stop it: 'short of having closed circuit TV'. Moreover, the mother positions herself as victim, enduring the suffering her son's behaviour causes: 'I can't trust any-body. That really irritates me.' At this point Chloe interrupts her mother to repeat, in almost every detail, the story of Steven's disregard for her property and the efforts she has made to protect her possessions.

After a long pause in the talk, the therapist again changes the subject. Turning to the mother, she asks about 'the arrangement w-with pocket money and stuff'. With this conversational manoeuvre she steers the conversation on to less contentious terrain, thus saving Steven's face, preserving the therapist's neutrality and avoiding the call for moral censure of Steven. However, once again, Chloe might hear the change of subject as evidence that the therapist has ignored, or is unconvinced by, her version of the troubles.

(Re)Formulations: the beginnings of therapist versions?

Formulations are conversational devices that appear to provide abstract and neutral summaries of what has just been said. They are easily recognized in everyday conversation as they are often prefaced by 'so what you seem to be saying is . . .' or 'so you think if . . .' However, formulations do more than simply summarize, they are also designed to 'package' preceding contributions to talk and 'prepare for future interaction' (Potter 1996: 48). This dual function is frequently visible, and exploited by therapists in conversation with families. That is, therapists utilize formulations to 'package' competing versions in an attempt to open up space for prospective non-blaming versions of the family's troubles. The next extract, a continuation of Extract 7.1, illustrates this in action.

Extract 7.3

Ch: I s'pose I'd agree with him they're better. Cos he doesn't (.) hit me. (1.5) It's just (.) he's start – (.) he always has gone in my room. But (.) he goes in (.) he used to know where I hid my purse. He's broken my stereo 'cos he took it on his paper round. And that was something someone bought me. Ehm. He'll just go in and take batteries out of things so he can use things. I came home last weekend and all my drawers were open. And I'd shut my door before I went out. And I knew he'd been in. He went in. And he roots through everything so he can find things. (2.0) And he just thinks there's nothing wrong with it. (2.0) To be rooting through all my private things 'cos now I've got my own room. (2.0)

Th: Did you used to share then?

Ch: I used to share with [sister].

Th: Right (2.0)

Ch: It's the biggest room and he wants it. (4.0)

Th: ((To Chloe and Steven)) So y-you (.) you've seen some improvements (.) so that y-you two aren't getting (.) physically into fights. But on the other hand (.) there's things that you're ((looks at Chloe)) not happy with at the moment.

Ch: Mm

After affirming the fact that she shared a bedroom with her sister, Chloe uses the new topic of 'the room' to further damage her brother's moral character: 'It's the biggest room and he wants it.' Chloe's utterance is met with a long pause in the conversation. This is followed by a faltering, hesitant delivery of the therapist's next turn: 'So y-you (.) you've seen some improvements.' This ignores Chloe's negative characterization of her brother in the previous turn and serves to cement the fact, constructed earlier in the talk, that Chloe and

Steven 'agree' that there have been some improvements. The therapist then becomes more specific about the changes for the better: 'so that y-you two aren't getting (.) physically into fights'. This redescription of the troubles, in contrast to Chloe's 'perpetrator–victim' categorization, implies that both Chloe and Steven may have been mutually responsible for the 'fights'. The second part of the therapist's turn – 'there's things that you're not happy with at the moment' – is artfully crafted to avoid any explicit moral evaluation of Steven, while at the same time making it clear to Chloe that her account of the troubles has been heard. To achieve this, the therapist employs a **rhetoric of deliberate vagueness**. Thus, Chloe's long and detailed list of her brother's alleged abuses is described as 'there's things', then minimized with 'you're not happy' and temporally relocated with 'at the moment'. Thus, the therapist's reformulation attenuates the power of Chloe's blaming version and saves Steven's face. The extract ends with Chloe's **minimal response token**, 'Mm'.

So we can see in this example that, with the deployment of certain conversational devices, therapists are able to ignore or mitigate blaming and hence avoid the implicit invitation to join in moral censure of individual family members. Therapists attempt to perform these discursive strategies while maintaining their impartiality. However, we have pointed out that there may be something of a paradox in these manoeuvres. There is some evidence that family members resurrect and strengthen their 'blaming' versions, believing that their previous attempts have not been sufficient to persuade the therapist of the veracity of their account of the troubles. We shall call this *the first paradox* of neutrality.

We now turn to the therapists' conversations with each other, 'behind the screen', and compare and contrast the management of competing versions in this context with therapists' strategies in their encounters with the family. Therapists' talk with their colleagues is organized by and oriented to the construction of acceptable 'therapist' versions of the troubles. These versions, as with the family versions, are achieved by drawing on similar conversational resources to family members and based on implicit and explicit practical–moral judgement by therapists of family members and their versions of the troubles. The analysis highlights how family therapists 'make knowledge' when they perform clinical judgements about families.

Making knowledge and performing clinical judgement: the second paradox

As the analysis above has shown, the therapist was faced with competing versions of the family troubles, which attributed accountability to particular parties. The mother's moral account of the troubles inculpated Chloe and Steven and depicted her as the victim of the unreasonable behaviour of both her children. In contrast, Chloe's version cast her as the victim of her brother's outrageous behaviour and blamed her mother for failing to intervene. In the following extract the therapists and the consultant can be heard working up the foundations for an accountability-neutral version of the family troubles that paradoxically relies on practical–moral evaluation of members and their versions.

Extract 7.4

Th: She (.) she *kept* on really about how (.) how he invades her privacy. And she was very tearful at times about that. At other times (.) she sort of seemed quite gleeful in how she allies herself with Mum, and upsetting him when she is able to do that. (2.0) I guess to acknowledge that from her point of view as well.

Con: Yeah. (2.0) I guess he must feel very isolated (1.5) in the family.

Th: Yeah I was thinking it's like they all have their point of view. They feel their pain and they're depressed about different things, aren't they?

Con: Mm yeah.

The extract opens with the therapist describing Chloe's account of her brother's unreasonable behaviour. The emphasis on 'she *kept* on' contains implicit evaluation of Chloe's telling of her brother's 'invasion of her privacy' and her presentation in the session, implying that Chloe's complaints about her brother were excessive and repetitive. The therapist then makes an observation about Chloe's emotional state at various points in her account of her brother's behaviour. That is, her apparent distress at certain times is contrasted with her 'quite gleeful' appearance at others. Moreover, in the therapist's formulation, Chloe's 'glee' is attributed to her successful alliance with her mother and how this results in 'upsetting' her brother. The complaints about her brother are, according to the therapist, sometimes consciously or deliberately used by Chloe to manipulate the relationship with her mother and brother. Thus, Chloe's version is ironized with this reference to **interest** or **stake**. In turn this ironization also implicitly mitigates the blame and moral censure, which Chloe's narrative of her brother's behaviour might otherwise have invited from the therapist and her colleagues. The therapist then ends with 'I guess to acknowledge that from her point of view'. This implies that while the therapy team may have made their own judgement on the sister's version of the troubles 'behind the screen', they must explicitly 'acknowledge' her apparent distress and complaints of victimization in the feedback to the family.

The consultant's next turn affirms the therapist's judgement about Chloe's telling of the troubles and what it reveals about family relationships. This sets up an identity 'in the making' for Steven, which depicts him as lonely and emotionally neglected as a result of being marginalized by the alliance between his mother and sister. This formulation has important moral connotations. It portrays Steven as victim, deserving sympathy and understanding, rather than as perpetrator of outrageous behaviour and thus deserving opprobrium. The therapist's next turn affirms this formulation and elaborates on it by depicting each family member as suffering, in different ways, for different reasons. This receives the consultant's endorsement at the next turn.

In this short extract we can see how the therapist and consultant collaborate in working up the seeds of an accountability-neutral, relational version of the troubles, in which all the family are victims and no one is to blame. In the talk that follows this extract the therapist and consultant go on to construct a more complete relational version of the troubles that attributes each member's individual private suffering to the father leaving the family. So, together, the therapist and consultant produce a meta-version of the troubles that artfully avoids them having to make any overt moral judgement about individual members and their respective versions. Thus, in one sense, their 'neutrality' is protected. However, paradoxically, to accomplish this they have had to make a series of covert, implicit moral judgements of members and their versions. We shall call this *the second paradox*. However, how will this work when the therapist returns to the family to deliver their formulation?

Moving from backstage to frontstage: the third paradox

How do the team's backstage versions of the troubles, with their inherent dependence on practical–moral evaluation, appear in the frontstage and how do therapists perform this 'public' feedback to families? By examining what happens in feedback, it can be shown that members are sensitive to therapist moral evaluation, however indirect, and that this is evident in the talk. Somewhat paradoxically, this data supports the contention that members are active in 'resisting' therapist attempts to construct versions which portray all members as morally adequate and blameless. We shall call this the *third paradox*. Moreover, therapists' accountability free versions sometimes result again in members reiterating their own, particular versions with their inherent attributions of blame and responsibility (they may resurrect the first paradox).

> **Extract 7.5**
> 1 Th: Ehm (.) I suppose some of the things I was struck with (.) and the
> 2 team as well is that (.) ehm I suppose it seemed like you were all
> 3 quite flat in some ways you know that you were all struggling
> 4 with maybe slightly different things. So I think you know I heard
> 5 loud and clear ((looks at mother)) you are struggling with the fact

6		that the children aren't getting on sometimes and ehm being the

6   that the children aren't getting on sometimes and ehm being the
7   only adult in the house thinking you know ((therapist laughs))
8   sometimes what's happening just feeling ground down by them
9   ehm and the fears about the future and perhaps you know if
10   Steven doesn't get his temper under control then (.) ehm (1.0)
11   and also stealing you know (.) you might think from time to time
12   it's just teenage but on the other hand you've got worries why
13   and how long will it go on for. And obviously Chloe saying really
14   quite clearly ((looks at Chloe)) you're fed up with your privacy
15   being invaded and Steven coming into your room and that being
16   difficult for you. (1.0) Also other things perhaps (1.0) feeling sad
17   about your dad not having much to say to you [and being] =
18 Ch: [I don't care]
19 Th: = Quite (.) at times but you know I guess those sorts of slightly
20   different perspectives. And then Steven really. I suppose we were
21   struck by how ((looks at Steven)) you might feel a bit out-
22   numbered really by the women in the family and feeling (.) ehm
23   perhaps you've lost various allies. Perhaps you feel you've lost
24   your father as an ally and perhaps like Steven in some ways feel-
25   ing a bit similar to his sister and she's now gone from the family
26   and also feel the same. Ehm and I thought Steven might also
27   share some of ((looks at mother)) your fears about will he be able
28   to control this in the future. Whether you ((looks at Steven)) will
29   be able to er not go down the road of losing his temper to get his
30   own way (.) so he might have some concerns about feeling like
31   lots of men have let him down he might feel they've let you
32   ((looks at mother)) down as well and in some way he has to make
33   up for that or be different or you know [bear some of that]
34 Mo: [Only one let me down]
35 Th: Ehm (.) the fact that you were able to come here. The fact you've
36   struggled on on your own really haven't you through many years
37   of difficult things happening and (1.0) then also the fact that
38   you've been able to come here and be very open. I think even
39   sometimes when you are on your own as a parent well (.) some-
40   times it can be even harder to let someone else in and see how
41   you're managing and what's happening. So that is very brave
42   really that you've all talked so openly [. . .]

Between lines 1 and 13, the therapist plants the seeds of the team's accountability-neutral version of the troubles, where all the family members are depicted as 'struggling' to cope with the loss of important relationships. The therapist also acknowledges, if equivocally, that she and the team have heard incommensurable versions ('different things') from each participant.

First, she rehearses the key blaming and mitigatory elements of the mother's version, artfully avoiding any blame or moral censure of Steven. However the therapist then moves to ironize subtly the mother's version by suggesting that *she*, not the therapist, may have nagging doubts about her normalization of the troubles. This opens up the space for alternative formulations – for example, the therapists' version – where the stealing could be constructed as deviant, and therefore as requiring managed change.

At line 13, the therapist turns to Chloe and summarizes her complaints and accusations against her brother, selecting out the least morally reprehensible aspects of the charges made: namely, Chloe's sense of her 'privacy being invaded' when her brother goes into her room. The charges of stealing, damaging personal belongings and verbal and physical intimidation made by Chloe in the family interview are deleted; as is the team's judgement that she may deliberately exaggerate her complaining to gain attention from her mother and distance her brother. Moreover, the emotional impact of her brother's behaviour on Chloe is minimized by the therapist (lines 14–16: 'you're fed up . . . and that being difficult for you').

Then, at lines 16–17, she attempts to assign affect to Chloe: 'also other things perhaps feeling sad about your dad not having much to say to you'. Thus, the therapist surreptitiously introduces a crucial theme in the therapists' formulation – the significance of the loss of the father – under the guise of Chloe's own version. However, at the next turn, talking over the therapist, Chloe disputes the claim that she is 'sad' about the lack of contact with her father. Indeed the attempted ascription by the therapist is refuted incisively (line 18: 'I don't care'). However, her 'resistance' is ignored by the therapist at the next turn, where further allusion is made to family members' competing versions (line 19: 'you know I guess those sort of slightly different perspectives').

Meeting with this dissent, the therapist moves to consider Steven's 'perspective' on the troubles. Steven made very little contribution to the talk in the session and did not offer a coherent, recognizable version. Consequently, the therapist (lines 20–26) draws on the case discussion 'behind the screen' to construct a morally adequate identity for Steven. Addressing him directly, the therapist tells a story of Steven's role in the troubles which positions him as 'victim'. The therapist also delivers the team's relational version, which depicts him as 'outnumbered . . . by the women in the family' and suffering the loss of 'various allies', namely his father and his oldest sister.

The therapist then turns to the mother, and adopting a rhetoric of deliberate vagueness, invokes an element of the mother's version to introduce the delicate issue of Steven's 'temper' (lines 26–30: 'I thought Steven might also share some of . . . your fears about will he be able to control this in the future . . . whether he will be able to ehm not go down the road of losing his temper to get his own way'). This implies that Steven is just as concerned as his mother about his 'temper' and his future ability to control it. This rhetorical manoeuvre, together with the ascription of the role of victim, ascribes a morally adequate identity to Steven.

Steven's moral identity receives more attention from the therapist in lines 30–33. The therapist, again drawing on the team's 'behind the screen' version, utilizes 'hyperbolic rhetoric' to portray him as 'let . . . down' by 'lots of men'. This not only further cements Steven in the role of victim, but opens up the space for the therapist to introduce the idea that he may be feeling burdened by the responsibility of having to be 'different' from, and feeling 'he has to make up' for, the various men who have 'let down' his mother. So this depicts Steven as morally responsible; dutifully endeavouring to compensate for all the men who have supposedly reneged on their commitment to the mother in the past. It also constructs him as unfairly and inappropriately saddling himself with this responsibility. However, at the next turn, the mother talks over the therapist, refuting the claim that lots of men have let her down (line 34: 'only one let me down'), which can be heard as an act of 'resistance' to the therapy team's formulation.

As before, when Chloe resisted the therapist's rhetoric of persuasion, the therapist does not acknowledge, or respond to, the mother's rebuttal. Instead, she continues with the delivery of her feedback to the family. First, she ascribes moral adequacy to the mother with a reformulation of key elements of the mother's version (lines 35–41). This is immediately followed by a positive, moral appraisal of all the family members (line 42: 'so that is very brave really that you've all talked so openly').

So the therapist's attempt to construct a commensurable, accountability-neutral version of the troubles, portraying them in relational terms, with each family member 'struggling' to come to terms with the 'loss' of significant relationships, met with resistance from family members. First Chloe attempts to refute the claim that she was 'feeling sad' about the lack of contact with her father. The second challenge to the therapist's relational formulation of the troubles comes from the mother when she corrects the therapist's claim that 'lots of men' have let her down. In both cases the therapist draws on the intrinsic inequalities in the conversational relationship to ignore the attempts at interjection and refutation and continues with the feedback from the team discussion.

Moreover, the extract shows that family members move to refute the therapist's claims when they detect some distortion or misrepresentation of their version of the troubles. The disputation of the therapist's feedback by Chloe arose when the therapist deviated from the rehearsal of Chloe's version to insert the claim that she was 'saddened' by the quality of her relationship with her father. Her interjection, and rebuttal of the claim that she 'cares' about this relationship, can be heard as an attempt to correct the therapist's inaccurate representation of her version. Similarly, the mother's interjection occurred at a point where the therapist was making the claim that 'lots of men' had let her and Steven down. The mother's turn, talking over the therapist, corrects what she hears as a misrepresentation of her version; that is, that the children's father is the sole cause of the troubles being experienced by the family.

This suggests that family members are oriented to any evidence of therapists 'mishearing' or 'misunderstanding' their versions, particularly when this has serious consequences for their attributions of accountability. For example, in the case of Chloe's resistance, the therapist's move to consider Chloe's relationship with her father shifted the focus away from the salient features of Chloe's version; that is, the maltreatment she alleges she is suffering at the hands of her brother and her efforts to persuade the therapist that Steven is to blame for all the troubles. Similarly, the mother's resistance to the therapist occurred when her version, primarily inculpating her ex-husband, was diluted by the therapist with the reference to 'lots of men'. This raises important questions about therapists' accountability-neutral versions. It seems likely, albeit somewhat paradoxically, that they might actually encourage resistance from family members. In other words, when therapists are doing 'neutrality' – that is, trying to avoid blaming and partiality to members' versions – family members may well detect that their version has not been heard. So, paradoxically, it seems that family members might sometimes feel moved to rebut therapists' attempts to construct them and their actions as morally adequate.

Summary

This chapter has concentrated on the discursive practices used by therapists engaged in the management of family members' competing versions in one case. The analysis of therapists' talk in interaction with the family in the 'front stage' showed how therapists have to negotiate the difficult balance of making members feel their versions have been heard, while also retaining a professional ethic of neutrality and impartiality. The analysis also demonstrated how therapists deploy certain devices, like a 'change of subject', in the management of contested realities and show a preference for the construction of relational (re)formulations of the troubles. However, we have also shown how by taking an interactional approach to neutrality and looking at what is actually said and done in therapy, we can reveal certain paradoxes, consequent upon 'doing neutrality', which are lost if we simply treat it as an ethic or motive. The three paradoxes are as follows.

1   In the performance of neutrality and in the effort to minimize blaming in the talk in interaction, devices such as changing the subject may subtly and indirectly reveal evaluation of members' versions. This may leave some members feeling that they have not been heard and cause them to try to convince the therapist by reiterating in stronger tones the blaming version they delivered earlier.

2   The analysis of therapists' conversation 'behind the screen' demonstrated how practical–moral judgements form the basis of the construction of a 'neutral' version of the troubles. The therapists' versions of the troubles were built upon the privileging of selected aspects of family members' accounts and the ironization of others.

3   When therapists attempt to deliver their accountability-neutral versions, family members seem sometimes to resist them, again seeing them as evidence of their own failure to convince the therapist of the veracity of their particular reading, or as evidence of the therapist's failure to grasp the point.

The three paradoxes of accountability-'neutral' versions might be understood if we recognize that therapists' versions can never really be 'neutral'. They are, and must be, constructed from the team's implicit and explicit practical–moral judgements of members, and their various versions. Thus, accountability-'neutral' versions must rely on selective hearings and reformulations of family members' stories about the troubles. These are resolutely acts of judgement and evaluation, of which family members *qua* members of society seem to be intuitively aware. Indeed, the turn by turn analysis demonstrated that family members are orienting to any sign, linguistic or paralinguistic, of therapist evaluation. In other words, they are 'prepared' to hear blame and responsibility in the therapist's talk.

In terms of everyday practice, the findings suggest that therapists need to be more aware and explicit about the practical–moral dimensions of their work. To family members, their versions, with all their inherent moralizing, really matter. Therefore, versions cannot be easily glossed in the search for 'a better story'. Families do not readily take up accountability-neutral, relational versions, no matter how artfully they are crafted. If, as we have suggested, neutrality is often illusory, then therapists need to look beyond the ubiquitous exhortations to 'side with everyone and no one'. They need mechanisms to engage with the ineluctably moral terrain in which they work.

While family therapy may be seen to be unusually morally laden and therefore not necessarily representative of other areas of clinical practice, there are similar issues at stake in many health and welfare encounters. We saw in Chapters 5 and 6 how saturated with practical moral judgements are domains like paediatrics and geriatrics. Child care social work and services concerned with people with mental health problems also entail moral judgement.

Even clinical genetics, with its probabilistic reasoning and relatively stable knowledge base, has to grapple with such matters. For example, there is a strong professional ethic of 'non-directiveness' in genetic counselling, which is proving quite thorny in practice, since people seeking genetic counselling often demand direction (*inter alia*, Clarke 1991, Wolff and Young 1995; Kessler 1997; Mitchie *et al.* 1997; van Zuuren 1997; Elwyn *et al.* 2000). It is to these and related matters that we turn in the final chapter, where we consider how we may be more realistic about clinical judgement in all its moral and social complexity, and how we may grapple with the implications in research, training and practice agendas.

8 Clinical judgement in context
Towards a more realistic realism

A fairly standard and not unreasonable response to a detailed sociological description of some small segment of the world is 'so what?'

(Strong 1979: 183).

In this book, we have described and illustrated a variety of ordinary and every-day clinical practices. We have tried to avoid making normative judgements about the practices we have illustrated, or at least we have tried to avoid making our opinions public. We have not, thus far, offered any clear prescriptions for practice. Our analytic ambitions have been more modest. Adopting a policy of 'ethnomethodological indifference' (Garfinkel and Sacks 1970), and suspending any presuppositions on what constitutes 'good' and 'bad' clinical judgement, our principal concern has been to show how judgement 'gets done' by ordinary practitioners, in mundane practice, in various health and welfare services. However, in taking this approach, we have potentially exposed ourselves to the 'so what?' question to which Strong refers above. In this chapter, we draw out some implications of our arguments, considering their relevance for research, practice and professional education and development. We begin the process by considering what we anticipate may be some of the principal counterarguments to our position.

Given the contemporary *zeitgeist*, we may anticipate some criticism from the leading proponents of EBP. We should note that, from clinicians in medicine, there has generally been a fairly balanced response to the possibilities offered by, and the limits of, experimentally based EBP. Medicine has been willing to accept and to argue publicly that many aspects of decision-making will always evade protocols and guidelines and that some judgements rely on individual expertise, 'humaneness' or patient choice (for example, Little 1995; Sackett *et al.* 1997; Elwyn and Gwyn 1999; Greenhalgh 1999). With one or two exceptions (for example, McNeish *et al.* 2002), the proponents of EBP in social care have tended to take a strong position against other ways of knowing and thinking, arguing that there are no really viable alternatives to experimentally based EBP, because these would rely on 'purely ideological assumptions and subjective views about the basis for decision-making' (Macdonald 1994: 405). By reviewing this strong position we have the opportunity to play devil's advocate to our own arguments and to build a response by considering what our approach has to offer.

We have argued principally that science, language, social interaction, history, emotion and moral judgement are important contextual elements in clinical judgement. In particular, we have stressed that when professionals produce accounts of people's symptoms or troubles they often perform important moral work, in the sense that they tell stories that are crafted locally to manage accountability. Often professionals confront multiple, and sometimes incommensurable, versions. These may be different inter-pretations of X-rays, or accounts of agency responsibility, or of who is respon-sible for a family's problems, or a child's symptoms. When they produce their case formulations carved from these competing versions of reality, clinicians depict differing degrees of certainty, seriousness, intent, responsibility and blameworthiness. We contend that ethnographic and discourse analytic work can be helpful in examining these intrinsic but neglected aspects of clinical judgement.

Although he does not present any empirical data, these arguments bear some relation to those advanced by Stephen Webb (2001) in the *British Journal of Social Work*. Webb takes issue with some of the claims made by proponents of EBP and particularly with their methodological exclusivity. He suggests that the tyranny of the RCT has led to the marginalization of more anthropological methods associated with interpretive social science, which can yield different understandings. The response to Webb's paper by Brian Sheldon, who is the founder of the Centre for Evidence-Based Social Services at the University of Exeter, provides the basis for our devil's advocate debate with our own position.

Sheldon's argument can be divided into a number of premises or proposi-tions as follows:

- *Proposition 1*. Pointing to the influence of history, culture, psychology and emotion in human reasoning processes undermines science and its products, leaving us prey to unsubstantiated, impassioned campaigns such as the parental lobby against the triple measles, mumps and rubella (MMR) vaccine. For Sheldon, science was designed as the remedy for these 'distorting tendencies' (Sheldon 2001: 802) and is insulated from them by its methodology and by its rigorous scepticism.
- *Proposition 2*. People who question evidence-based approaches operate with a crude understanding of science and see it as applying only in physics, chemistry or biology. This proposition has a

corollary: proponents of evidence-based approaches know what science is and what it is not.

- *Proposition 3.* We must beware of relaxing the hierarchy of evidence, as this will lead to unsafe practices – the same criteria of reliability and validity should be transferable from biomedicine, or indeed the airline industry, to other domains of human service activity.
- *Proposition 4.* Deduction produces better and more reliable products than induction. Sheldon notes: 'Mention "maternal deprivation", "attachment theory", or "moral development" on a social work training course and you will get Pavlovian reflex citations of Bowlby and Salter-Ainsworth (1965) and Piaget (1958). Great historical figures, interesting theories, but decades of more careful *empirical* work has changed the picture very substantially' (Sheldon 2001: 803).
- *Proposition 5.* Evidence-based approaches can immunize staff against famous or fashionable ideas by showing them the truth. A number of examples are given for this, including the following: 'The popular idea (who dared challenge it?) that child sexual abuse was absolutely rampant in Britain in the 1980s, fed by bad medicine, and politically inspired feminist methodology, led to the catastrophes at Cleveland and Orkney . . . I propose that evidence-based training, supervision, management and practice are the most promising correctives to all this' (Sheldon 2001: 804).
- *Proposition 6.* Sociological and anthropological approaches must be handled with care, because they do not produce really useful knowledge, are often driven by theory or dogma and have the tendency to confuse 'close familiarity and favourite theories with cultural fact' (Sheldon 2001: 806).

If Sheldon's propositions are correct then a great deal of what we have argued in this book may be subject to criticism. For example, we have repeatedly asserted the social, interactional, interpretive and emotional nature of a good deal of professional activity and indeed of science itself, we have argued for the practical utility of the inductive methods associated with sociological and anthropological approaches in understanding some of the contexts and forms of knowledge that frame what professionals do and we have suggested that the concept of evidence-based practice needs to be broadened to include such methodologies. In order to defend and clarify our position, we provide a response to some of Sheldon's arguments below. However, first, we want to move towards a rapprochement and consider some points of agreement.

First, we agree with Sheldon's arguments about the problems with theory-driven observations. In Chapter 4 we illustrated the ways in which theory, particularly in its simplified handbook form, can affect case formulation in very significant ways. There is indeed a risk that favoured ideas finish up constituting the things they are supposed to describe. We observe the interaction between a mother and infant armed with our attachment checklist and – Eureka – we find an attachment disorder. In our view, 'The only theory worth having is that which you have to fight off, not that which you speak with profound fluency' (Hall 1992: 280). We can only 'fight off' theory if we can see its distorting effects as well as its practical utility. We return to this point in due course. Second, we agree that disciplined inquiry is important in any professional context. Although we do not read Webb's arguments as an apology for ad hocery, he does talk about *'abandoning'* (Webb 2001: 76), rather than supplementing, mechanistic and experimental approaches, and thereby may leave himself open to the criticism that he is throwing out the baby with the bathwater. On this basis, Sheldon may be right to point out that Webb's argument could be read as an overoptimistic defence of professional artistry, in that he does not explicitly provide any suggestions about how the methods he advocates may be deployed in a practice context. We attend to this omission in due course (see also Taylor and White 2000). However, beyond these points of agreement, Sheldon's position is deeply problematic and we must correct some serious misrepresentations in his arguments.

Misunderstanding science: why we don't need the 'science wars'

Sheldon's arguments in defence of science are unnecessary. Breathing life and culture into science does not undermine it as an enterprise, nor does it devalue its products (Latour 1999). In this book, we have treated certain aspects of clinical judgement as everyday science, but have shown how these rely a great deal on interpretive skills and on ideas about what can reasonably be known at a given time about a given condition. Sheldon seems to aspire to emotionless reason, equating affect with error. Through this emotionless reason we may, he suggests, reach conditions of relative certainty. Nowhere does he depict the tentative science of the esoteric domain that we considered in Chapter 4. Nowhere does he acknowledge the intrinsic role of emotion in human reasoning. While he concedes that they may be open for revision, for Sheldon science delivers clear *answers* to pressing practice problems. He uses analogies from dentistry and the airline industry to ironize Webb's arguments in favour of human creativity:

> For all I know there may be dentists . . . who base their practice on
> *Zen and the Art of Root Canal Work*, but if there are, I wager one would
> have little trouble getting an early appointment . . .

When we the middle class buy services, travel across the Atlantic say, or have our brake pipes replaced, then we become card carrying positivists. Thought experiment:

> This is your flight facilitator speaking, sorry for the delay everyone but we are still waiting for the flip charts to come aboard. As soon as we have attained this and established a genuine consensus on course heading and purpose of travel we shall be on our way.
>
> (Sheldon 2001: 807)

While these are artful linguistic strategies on Sheldon's part, they carry two implicit and unsupportable propositions. First, they assume that flying aircraft or drilling teeth are similar activities to, for example, deciding whether someone is lying about their child's injury, is able to tolerate the stress of caring for their terminally ill partner, really wants to be tested for Huntington's disease or has properly understood one's messages about safe sex. This is patently not the case. Second, they assume that positivism and the experimental methodologies associated with it are the only properly rigorous means of inquiry. Other methods become necessary evils that we will have to tolerate in some practice domains until appropriate experimental designs have been produced.

Sheldon's reading of science is as a realm of certainty that can protect the public from professional vagueries. He claims privilege for this reading since, as a member of the evidence-based practice movement, he 'believes' in science and this apparently qualifies him to define it. Whither the tentative and creative science of the laboratory described by Fleck (himself a scientist)? Whither the embodied reasoning of Damasio (himself a scientist)? They have no place in Sheldon's EBP. That is why he is stranded in his own interminable science war. Invigorating science does not amount to a denial of its value, or of the existence of reality. Neither does it signal the end of disciplined research, or the beginning of 'methodological anarchy' (Clavarino *et al.* 1995: 225). These kinds of accusations are seriously misplaced, as Latour notes:

> Once there is no longer a mind-in-a-vat looking through the gaze at an outside world the search for certainty becomes less urgent, and thus there is no great difficulty in reconnecting with the relativism, the relations, the relativity on which the sciences have always thrived ... there is no great difficulty in recognizing the human character of scientific practice, its lively history, its many connections with the rest of the collective. Realism comes back like blood through the many vessels now reattached by the clever hands of the surgeons – there is no longer any need for a survival kit. After following this

route, no one would even think of asking the bizarre question 'Do you believe in reality?'

(Latour 1999: 16–17)

Latour is fond of using arterial metaphors to humanize science. He is captivated by science in this flowing, circulatory, human form. With this celebratory definition, who needs the science wars? Certainly not Latour's contemporary scientist subjects. They appear as large as life, smiling from the photographs in his books – and not a weapon in sight.

So why is Sheldon's science so sure of itself? Sheldon treats science as though it were entirely reducible to the hypothetico-deductive method. He is exclusively concerned with testing the validity of what is already known, or at least has already been thought about. This is why he prefers deduction to induction. If we start from a falsifiable hypothesis and pare down our questions accordingly, we may indeed produce a single answer to our question. Of course, this activity can have considerable value – it is the mainstay of RCTs – but its value depends on the appropriateness of the question and, without inductive reasoning, there would quite simply be few ideas to test. Moreover, professional practice is itself often dependent on inductive reasoning, as Downie and Macnaughton note:

> The concept of evidence, as it is used by scientists, is logically related to that of an hypothesis. Information, data, observations and experiments become 'evidence' when they are for or against a specific hypothesis ... The concept of evidence as used by detectives, or forensically differs in two respects: the data and observations *suggest* a hypothesis ... about a specific or particular state of affairs. The concept of evidence that applies to *medical research* is like that of the scientist, and the concept that applies to *clinical consultations* is like that of the detective.
>
> (Downie and Macnaughton 2000: 183)

Thus, both induction and deduction, often as part of a productive, recursive process, are important aspects of knowledge production. Without induction there would be no inquiry. Someone first has to think of something, or serendipitously discover a phenomenon that needs explaining. What has not been thought about and conceptualized simply 'is'. It is part of the tacit dimension – something no one notices – or it is an enigma that everyone knows about, but no one can understand or explain. We cannot promise to do very much about the enigma problem, but we argue below that we may be able to suggest some possibilities for interrogating the taken for granted.

Can EBP provide protection from fashion and fad?

In our view, Sheldon is on his shakiest terrain when he asserts that evidence-based approaches could have prevented events like the Cleveland scandal (Butler-Sloss 1988). In the 1980s in Cleveland (UK) a large number of children were removed from their families because of suspected sexual abuse. The principal evidence in their cases was not a disclosure from the children, but a since discredited diagnostic procedure ('reflex anal dilatation') that was much in favour at the time with a local paediatrician, Dr Marietta Higgs. The theory was that if a child's anus dilated in response to the test, they had been subject to sexual abuse. This now seems a preposterous assertion, but at the time Higgs's persuasive rhetoric, presumably invoking all kinds of scientific evidence, was sufficiently potent to persuade members of the judiciary to grant court orders in respect of the children. This took place at a time when population figures for sexual abuse in childhood as high as one in four were routinely invoked to justify such interventions (Lloyd 1992). Sheldon thinks that EBP would have prevented this. We wonder how. It is notoriously difficult to produce population indices on the prevalance of child sexual abuse, or to falsify existing claims, however counterintuitive they may appear. Even if reliable epidemiological data were available, how would it be possible to rule out the possibility that a frenzied paedophile was operating in the area? EBP would certainly have provided social workers and medics with a training in scepticism, which is a necessary but insufficient criterion for good decision-making. Sheldon is disparaging of the validity and reliability of anthropological and discourse analytic methods, and subtly equates them with the abyss of relativism, but it is precisely these methods that can unmask 'fashion and fad'.

For example, during the 1970s it was very fashionable for ENT consultants to remove the tonsils and adenoids of their younger patients. Michael Bloor's (1976) ethnographic study of eleven outpatient clinics showed wide variation in practices and in the typifications of their patients' problems produced by different specialists. We cannot claim that Bloor's study was responsible for the subsequent change in practice, but had policy-makers bothered to read it, it may have raised some interesting questions about some of the more arbitrary aspects of business as usual in ENT clinics. More specifically in relation to the Cleveland crisis, we have shown in Chapter 5 that child welfare professionals (at least in the UK) continue to prefer to hear children's versions of family troubles as true and to cast doubt on adult accounts, and so to inculpate parents. Moreover, White's (1997b) ethnographic study of child care social work, a decade after Cleveland picked out exactly social workers' fears of questioning the dominant ideas about sexual abuse to which Sheldon refers. She notes:

> It is . . . hazardous [for social workers] to dispute the truism 'believe the child'. The competent individual will whisper their doubts in corners, will swear the accomplice to secrecy. Since the mid to late 1980s (when social work involvement in cases of child sexual abuse increased), I can recall hearing this orthodoxy explicitly challenged only once or twice.
>
> (White 1997b: 195)

However, while social workers normally privilege the child's voice, a child's account is less likely to be believed if they are asserting that all is well at home, when social workers' suspicion has been aroused that it is not, either by a referral or by a previous statement from the child. Under these circumstances, the scepticism usually reserved for parental versions is reinstated and the child's account loses its privileged status. Clearly, this may often be absolutely the right way to proceed to protect children, but the taken-for-granted assumption about its intrinsic, always and forever correctness can make allegations of sexual abuse virtually incorrigible – which is precisely what happened with some of the cases in Cleveland.

At a more micro level, Lloyd (1992) used conversation analysis to study the linguistic practices of therapists and social workers in the USA, when they were conducting forensic interviews with children in cases of suspected sexual abuse. His data illustrate how denials from children that abuse had taken place were dispreferred by the adult interviewers, who would respond to such denials with subtle censure or with further questions. Lloyd summarizes his findings as follows:

> The adults elicit children's confirmations by producing candidate response initiations [suggesting the answer], ratifying confirming turns, censuring children's non-confirming responses, producing subsequent versions of initiations [suggesting the answer again] and treating children's weak agreements as strong agreements.
>
> (Lloyd 1992: 109)

The techniques in vogue at the time for eliciting children's disclosures were dramaturgical. They involved the use of puppets and play acting. The following is an example of an adult censuring a child for producing a non-confirming response:

(Adult treats Nicole as animating the Houndy puppet)

Adult: Do you remember that part?
Child: No I don't
Adult: Oh Houndy. You were doing so good. I think you're losing your memory. How about . . .

> (Lloyd 1992: 115)

Lloyd is at pains to point out that he is not passing judgement on whether abuse had actually taken place; like us he adopts a policy of 'indifference'. However, his data illustrate perfectly the local reproduction of certain ideas that were dominant at the time, and were treated by practitioners working with sexual abuse as the only right and proper way to think. Thus, Sheldon is mistaken on two counts. First, he gives no adequate account of how EBP in its current incarnation may have prevented Cleveland; second, he fails to recognize the value of sociological inquiry in rendering the taken for granted explicit, or making it strange, and therefore open to debate and challenge.

Sociological inquiry: some uses and abuses

Sheldon is deeply suspicious of sociology. He equates the discipline with grand theory, particularly Marxism, which had a significant impact on social work in the 1970s, but produced 'no positive advice about what we might actually *do* about child abuse or mental health care' (Sheldon 2001: 804). Perhaps the advocates of the 'strong' evidence-based programme have no place for the social, but from where we sit, clinical work is intrinsically interactional and is saturated with moral and cultural influences. If we are properly to understand their impact we need some analytic tools to help us to interrogate them. We agree that the crude version of structural Marxism that affected social work in the 1970s is not perhaps the most promising candidate, but as we noted in Chapter 3, discourse analysis and the sociology of everyday life meet the job specification very nicely.

Sheldon pays scant regard to interpretive social science. He concedes that 'anthropological' approaches have some value but raises serious concerns about reliability and validity in such studies. This is despite a vast sociological literature attending to just these matters (for an accessible summary see Murphy *et al.* 1998: 167–98; Silverman 1993: 197–211). It is unsurprising that sociologists, anthropologists and discourse analysts have themselves been concerned to ensure the quality of their work. It is an advisable strategy for anyone interested in their own occupational survival. The criteria for judging qualitative research may be different in some ways from those applied to quantitative work, but they are rigorous nevertheless. For example, the researcher may ensure that they have examined any negative or atypical cases that arose during data analysis to ensure that competing explanations of the phenomenon under question are explored, that they have been transparent about their methods of data collection and analysis, that they have undertaken simple counting of the frequency of certain events and that they have used detailed verbatim extracts or have kept contemporaneous fieldnotes. A few suspect experimental studies that involve, for example, woefully inadequate samples, concealed by impressive looking charts and tables, do not in any way shake the validity of rigorous RCTs, and neither does the existence of poor quality interpretive work in any way undermine the value of disciplined qualitative inquiry.

So what kinds of qualitative work may be useful to professionals? We have shown examples throughout the book of detailed ethnographic work and we say a little more about how these studies and the methods associated with them may be used in day-to-day practice in due course. However, we should first consider some potential violations of what we consider to be the most cherished principles of qualitative methodologies. By far the greatest blights on the interpretive landscape are what Silverman calls 'naive' interview studies. He notes:

> How could anybody think that what we ought to do is to go out into the field to report people's exciting, gruesome or intimate experiences? . . . Naive interviewers believe that the supposed limits of structural sociology are overcome by an open-ended interview schedule and a desire to catch authentic experience.
>
> (Silverman 1993: 199)

These studies often take an 'underdog' perspective (Murphy *et al.* 1998: 193), situating the researcher on the side of the oppressed, predefined, of course, by the researcher often using simplistic versions of feminism or Marxism. These studies have been overrepresented in research in the health and social care fields, where, for example, doctors are typically presented as oppressors and patients as oppressed. We were critical of this kind of study in Chapter 3 and have avoided citing any work of this kind in this book. However, this refusal easily to take sides (some sides are worth taking, but this is a matter for the conscience) and fight the good fight should not be confused with stasis and inertia. We have adopted the view that qualitative studies which describe in detail how clinicians do what they do can have transformative potential (Bloor 1997; Silverman 1997), which is a point we develop further below.

How individual clinicians go about creatively 'making sense' of cases, how they arrive at knowledge claims about situations they confront, how case formulations evolve and how clinical decision-making 'gets done' have not previously been viewed as salient issues by the advocates of EBP. The processes of clinical judgement and case formulation require clinicians to make knowledge as well as use it (Taylor and White 2000). This involves creative, rhetorical–moral practices and cannot be reduced to a technical–rationalist exercise where clinicians decide how to proceed by referring to a codified body of formal knowledge. Therefore, one key implication of our arguments is that, at best, the evidence-based approach will only ever be able to provide partial answers to the mundane clinical and moral dilemmas faced by practitioners operating in the hurly burly of modern health and social care agencies.

Of course, clinicians are obliged to be realists in their encounters with patients or clients. They have to get real things done. However, in so doing they are also obliged to construct versions of events and to use a whole range of cognitive, analytic, linguistic, interpretive, imaginative and emotional resources. Perhaps, then, at the sharp end of practice, we are, as Hall (1997: 240) suggests, 'obliged to be realists, constructivists and constitutive', all at once! We think that this more relative reading of clinical judgement is, paradoxically, more realistic than the naive realism promoted by EBP (Latour 1999). So how may the definition of EBP be widened to include more descriptive studies and how may these be put to use in research, professional practice and education?

Connecting research with the swampy lowlands of practice

The current approach to understanding the relationship between research and policy/practice is roughly synonymous with what Silverman and Gubrium (1989) call the 'state-counsellor' model and Bryant (1991) terms the 'social engineering' model. Bryant describes the social engineering model as follows:

> The customer or client wants information about, or an analysis of, something, and the [social scientist] is contracted to provide it. The customer has an objective and the [social scientist] helps to engineer it by using expertise in research design and techniques to obtain relevant information and by drawing upon the stock of [social scientific] knowledge in order to advise how it might best be achieved.
>
> (Bryant 1991: 177)

While, as we have noted, this model can have considerable utility and is appropriate for some research questions, many of the issues that practitioners face and much of their professional activity have limited tractability in relation to a top-down applied science model. In this book we have examined the utility of an alternative model of applied social science that may fruitfully be employed as part of a more inclusive version of EBP. There is a pressing need for health and social care services to embrace a dialogical approach to the relationship between research and practice. The dialogical model is derived from the work of Giddens (e.g. 1987), and three propositions underpin the approach.

1   Social research is intrinsically contestable. Therefore, it cannot always be applied in a top-down linear manner, but has to be linked to the potential for persuading actors to understand, challenge and expand

the forms of knowledge upon which they draw in their mundane activities.

2   The mediation and transformation of cultural settings by social research can be as important as establishing generalizations.

3   One of the most significant contributions social science can make is to encourage 'communication via research, of what it is like to live in one cultural setting to those in another' (adapted from Giddens 1987: 47).

Taylor and White (2000) propose that discursive approaches afford the opportunity for just this kind of dialogue by creating a union between the 'high ground' of research and the 'swampy lowlands' of practice (Schön 1983, 1987). By grounding the specifics of practice in the detail of talk-in-interaction, it becomes possible to examine the local, contingent consequences of a given form of practice or particular technique. For example, in Chapter 7 we showed that it was possible to analyse the local relevance of therapist feedback of 'neutral' versions. This demonstrated, somewhat counterintuitively, that one of the local, real-time consequences of this mundane practice can be resistance from family members who want to pre-suade the therapist of the veracity of their own individual blaming versions. Thus, as we have already argued, analyses of this kind are capable of exposing how practice differs from idealized, theoretically driven accounts of process. However, they can also lead to challenge and revision of theory, to accommodate findings grounded in and emergent from mundane practice. Thus, in this regard, discourse-analytic work could act as a 'bridge' between research and practice, with research and practice in a mutual and recursive dialogue. This holds the promise of a research agenda less alienated from the key issues of practice and practitioners more actively involved in research.

Developing reflexivity: beyond reflection on action

At the start of this book we pointed to the deficits in Donald Schön's concept of professional artistry. It offered no means by which the 'tacit dimension' could be made visible, reportable and therefore accountable and subject to debate. It is our contention that the kinds of studies we have used in this book can be deployed to this end, as part of professional education, supervision and development. For example, simply reading ethnographies about ourselves can help us to examine, more self-consciously and analytically, what we are thinking about and doing in our professional practice. This does not mean that we will necessarily want to change anything. We might want to debate, or to change some things some of the time, but we might even feel rather proud of other bits. However, we can only make these judgements once we have developed a particular kind of orientation to our routines and practices. In social science, this kind of orientation is generally referred to as 'reflexivity', which differs in particular ways from the more familiar concept of 'reflection'.

Reflexivity is a slippery term and there is considerable ambiguity and variety in the way it is interpreted (Taylor and White 2000). It is often treated as synonymous with 'reflection', which we may see as a form of 'benign introspection' (Woolgar 1988: 22): a process of looking *inward*, and thinking about how our own life experiences or significant events may have impacted upon our thinking, or upon the research or assessment process. As we noted in Chapter 1, this form of reflection has been influential in nursing and social work, and typically involves the practitioner keeping confessional diaries. We have noted that there is a danger with this kind of reflection, that we learn little about the encounter itself and a great deal about the struggles and torments of the practitioner. While this kind of reflection is a good deal better than failing to think at all about what one is saying, writing or doing, in promoting the concept of reflexivity we advocate a rather different reading. We want to interpret and apply the concept of reflexivity to denote the kind of destabilization or problematization of taken-for-granted knowledge and day-to-day reasoning that we have repeatedly referred to in this book. Treated in this way, reflexivity becomes a process of looking *inward* and *outward*, to the social and cultural artefacts and forms of thought that saturate our practices. In support of this argument we make a distinction between different levels of reflective and reflexive practice and illustrate the potential value of ethnographic and discourse analytic work at each level.

From practising reflectively to practising reflexively

Reflection-on-action can be defined as 'making sense of an action after it has occurred and possibly learning from the experience which extends one's knowledge base' (Eraut 1994: 146). As we noted above, this idea has spawned the reflective practice movement in nursing and social work. We argued in Chapter 1 that the problem with these is that they simply present professional activity within the boundaries of what is assumed to be the right and proper way to think. That is, they use tacit knowledge, but they do not examine its influence. Similarly, most clinical supervision and case discussions or presentations are characterized by this type of reflection. In these settings practitioners may be said to be 'practising reflectively'.

Clearly, the augmentation of these traditional methods for 'reflection-on-action' with ethnographic and discourse analysis would be of some value. For example, the production of audio and video recordings and verbatim transcripts of talk in various settings would have the effect of 'slowing down the action', and might make it possible for clinicians to make audible/visible phenomena that would not be available in real-time analyses. As Elwyn and Gwyn note,

> there is much more depth to be explored in the process of com-
> munication, and the tools normally used are insufficient to examine
> the layers of meaning that lie within the text of exchanges. The
> microanalysis of talk can inform the essence of medical practice,
> define principles for effective communication, attach meanings to a
> patient's story, as well as help doctors share ideas about fears and
> hopes for the future.
>
> (Elwyn and Gwyn 1999: 186)

That is, discursive methods would create greater opportunities for 'making sense of an action' and 'learning from experience'. Broadly, then, it offers a method for developing our understanding of the conversational worlds of health and welfare practice. As such it can play a valuable role in clinical training and supervision, in that it provides practitioners with the tools with which to practise reflexively. For example, in contemporary family therapy theory and practice, recognition of the importance of the therapist's contribution to what is observed and discussed in therapy has led to much greater emphasis on the therapist as participant as well as observer. In this context, the routine discursive analysis of mundane practice would provide the means of exploring the inherent tensions associated with being both participant and observer and enable therapists to develop and maintain some form of 'self-reflexivity'. Thus, at this level, it might accomplish a shift from practising reflectively to practising reflexively. However, as a mere adjunct to more orthodox approaches, and while operating within the constraints of fads, fashions or theoretical presuppositions, such forays into reflexivity may be prematurely foreclosed, before they in any way defamilarize what practitioners have ceased to question.

From practising reflexively to practising reflexivity

We have argued that interpretive social science lends itself to the examination of clinical judgements, decision-making and use of knowledge claims in individual cases. Thus, it offers a way of interrogating the institutional practices and specialist knowledges of particular domains and how they are put to work in mundane practice. The benefit of the detailed, sequential analysis of talk-in-interaction in health and social care settings is that it can sensitize practitioners to 'listening' rather than 'doing'. By this we mean paying greater attention to our own constituting practices as well as those of our clients and patients to help us to achieve greater critical distance from our routinized practices. For example, the analysis of the 'taken-for-granted', normative notions of 'best practice' in family therapy presented in Chapter 7 showed that these practices can sometimes have unintended and unwanted consequences. In this way, discursive analyses of actual practice can expose the deficiencies of received professional wisdom and formal textbook knowledge. The concepts and methods associated with discourse analysis and ethnography can be used by practitioners themselves to make sense of how they use and produce knowledge in day-to-day practice. As Taylor and White (2000: 201) conclude, 'since we cannot escape these processes of knowledge making, it is important to understand them better'. Discursive analysis is a means of understanding them better and so provides a way of practising reflexivity.

In sum, 'practising *reflexively*' would start with listening more carefully to our clients and patients, the different versions of cases and how they are constituted in interaction in service settings. 'Practising *reflexivity*' can only start when we begin listening more carefully to ourselves, attending to our rhetorics of persuasion and our own constituting practices; that is, listening with a critical ear to our sense-making and knowledge-making practices. How would this affect professional education and development?

Beyond training: educating judgement

In making their case for 'humane medicine', Downie and Macnaughton (2000) put forward a number of ideas about medical education that we find compelling and think are transferable to other health and welfare professions. We also think we can usefully supplement their proposals using our own approach. Downie and Macnaughton stress the importance of interpretive ability and insight. For this, they argue, doctors need not just training, but a broad *education*. Training may deliver technical competence, and we all want technically competent doctors. This would be sufficient if doctoring required only technical skill or craft knowledge. Downie and Macnaughton dispute this (see also Greenhalgh and Hurwitz 1999; Launer 1999). They argue that, unlike carpentry or engineering, the humaneness of doctoring renders it intrinsically moral. Some of the moral questions can be addressed through ethics teaching, but the authors argue that this can never bring moral matters to life in the way the arts can. To this end they distinguish between education and training (Peters 1966), arguing that the former denotes a broadening of vision, a liberating, a widening out, and the latter a focusing in on some specific technical competency, such as taking blood. Education ideally provides heuristic devices that have broad applicability and allow the recipient to make connections to other disciplines. It produces an openness to ideas and to the possibilities of change. In fact, education has intrinsic value and should bring about positive change. Obviously not all students will achieve this, but those who can should have the opportunity to release their minds. While recognizing that we want our doctors to be trained as well as educated, Downie and Macnaughton argue that:

> Doctors through a combination of excessive busyness and solidarity, can easily lose their broad perspectives to become, not just work-aholic, but blinkered to the point of not knowing *when* to use their medical skill – although they might know very well *how* . . . Hence it is important for the humane doctor to have, not only ethical sensitivity, but a broad perspective on life. This is necessary to ensure humane judgement.
>
> (Downie and Macnaughton 2000: 169)

A similar point is made by Greenhalgh and Hurwitz:

> At its most arid, modern medicine lacks a metric for existential qualities such as inner hurt, despair, hope, grief and moral pain that frequently accompany, and often indeed constitute, the illnesses from which people suffer. The relentless submission during the course of medical training of skills deemed 'scientific' – those which are eminently measureable but unavoidably reductionist – for those that are fundamentally linguistic, empathic and interpretive should be seen as anything but a successful feature of the modern curriculum.
>
> (Greenhalgh and Hurwitz 1999: 48)

To foster and retain the broad perspective, Downie and Macnaughton suggest a series of 'special study modules', to include the humanities, philosophy and other components of educatedness. Assessment in these modules, they suggest, may involve writing an essay on the protrayal of doctors in Ibsen's plays and considering what doctors can learn from a study of these works. This kind of imaginative teaching can help to move professionals towards practising reflexivity, since it exposes them to different ways of representing what they do, and thereby may create some critical distance and crucially foster openness and breadth.

We find these ideas appealing, but suggest that it may be even more useful for students in health and welfare to learn to interrogate their own stories as texts. This is no substitute for the dissemination of formal knowledge, but it is, we suggest, an essential addition to the curriculum. Students need to absorb knowledge, but they then need to interrogate how they use it and what they add to it and take away. Using transcripts of naturally occurring conversation, for example, students may be encouraged to look at how formal knowledge gets used in practice, how it interacts with moral reasoning and what the relationship is between certainty and uncertainty. They may thus, in due course, make recordings of their own practice and use them for reasoned debate (for further examples of and exercises in the practical application of discourse analytic techniques, see Taylor and White 2000).

This is particularly important in those occupations that rely to a large extent on the exoteric knowledge of the broader languaging community. Obvious examples are social work and therapeutics. In these sectors there is a real danger that the apparent certainties produced by the uncritical use of this popular knowledge prematurely foreclose alternative readings of cases (see Chapter 4). For example, in our experience, these professions often operate with a very negative view of the role of biology or organic pathology in some of the problems they confront, with frequent perjorative references to the 'medical model'. Yet, as Launer notes in the context of family therapy:

> To make the assumption that biology is a naively determinist frame-work for seeing the world and to profess disdain for such a powerful and widely accepted discourse about how the world functions is to identify oneself as uninterested in one of the main cultural streams of our time.
>
> (Launer 2001: 166)

Students and practitioners should be encouraged to generate alternative readings of their cases and properly consider them. While this is pressing in these 'social' domains, reflexivity remains important in other areas. In Chapter 6, we showed the range of warrants used by a paediatrician in one case. This is not unusual. Chapters 4 and 5 showed how the voices of science and morality interlock in many settings.

In this book, we have urged you to be realistic about clinical judgement and to see it in its complexity. We have urged a scepticism about some of the simplistic demands of policy-makers and the unrealistic claims emanating from certain factions of the evidence-based practice movement. The ideals of reason and progress through dispassionate inquiry were laudible aims of modernity. As Bruno Latour notes, they were 'for many decades our most cherished source of light, defended by giants, before [they] fell to the care of dwarfs' (Latour 1999: 300). In our view, the dwarfs are fast colonizing clinical judgement, which demands reason, emotion and, most of all, an intelligence that is disciplined *and* creative. It is time to revitalize science by adding emotion. To this end, we have not told you how to produce better case for-mulations. Instead, we have shown you some examples of clinicians doing judgements. We have done so in order to encourage you to build your own realistic ethics. As Foucault observes:

> People have to build their own ethics, taking as a point of departure the historical analysis, sociological analysis, and so on that one can provide for them. I don't think that people who try to decipher the

truth should have to provide ethical principles or practical advice at the same moment, in the same book and the same analysis. All this prescriptive network has to be elaborated and transformed by people themselves.

(Foucault 1994: 132)

People cannot do this, however, while their presuppositions and shortcuts remain taken for granted. By using detailed ethnographic and discourse analytic data as part of a dialogical model of applied social science, an inclusive EBP and a broad and continuing professional education, clinicians can be helped to see the process of judgement more realistically, and hence may become more reflexive, analytic and systematic in their sense-making activities. By attending to *how work gets done*, rather than to how it *should* be done, we hope this book forms the basis for fruitful dialogue between research and practice.

Appendix
Transcription conventions

The following transcription symbols are commonly used in conversation analysis.

[ ]	overlapping talk
//	onset of overlapping talk
( )	inaudible, and hence untranscribed, passage
(talk)	uncertainty about the transcription
((laughs))	contextual information not transcribed as actual sounds heard
(0.8)	pauses timed in tenths of second
(.)	audible, but very short pause
talk or talk	italics or underlining indicate emphasis
TALK	upper case indicates loudness in comparison to surrounding talk
tal–	abrupt end to utterance
>slow<	noticeable slowing of tempo of talk
=	latching of utterances
–	a dash marks a sudden end to an utterance
::	colons mark a prolonged syllable or sound
.h	laughter (or, without full-stop, an outbreath)

Glossary

Authorization procedures: this refers to the strategies by which speakers or writers seek to establish the authenticity of their version of events.

Accounts and accounting practices: these are versions of events produced by participants in encounters. The concept of 'accounts' is derived from *ethnomethodology*, which argues that all social action involves both an act (or an utterance) and a subsequent (or prospective) account of that act. Accounts *of* events also usually embody some kind of account or justification *for* the action taken. The justification offered will depend on the context in which the talk is taking place. Thus, what people say cannot be taken as an unproblematic reflection of what really happened.

Bayes' theorem: a mathematical formula used clinically to calculate the probability that a member of a given population who has a given symptom also has a given disease. It is in common use in many areas of practice, particularly clinical genetics and epidemiology.

Blamings: this term is used here to refer to attributions of responsibility for causing particular problems. It does not necessarily imply malicious intent.

Category bound activities: see *membership categorization*.

Contrast structures: derived from the work of Dorothy Smith (1978), these are two-part sequences in talk or text, in which the first part of a statement sets up expectations, and the second signals deviation from these 'norms'. Contrast structures are a powerful way of marking deviance in talk.

Conversation analysis: grew from *ethnomethodology's* focus on the detail of what people actually do. Using detailed transcripts, conversation analysis focuses on the sequential features of talk. That is, the turns people take, the pauses in the talk, the way new topics are introduced and so forth.

Decision analysis: adapts *Bayes' theorem* by adding calculations of the 'utility', or risks and benefit, of a treatment.

Deduction/deductive reasoning: hypothesis or theory driven research that generally sets out to test ideas, rather than generate them (contrast with *induction/inductive reasoning*).

Definitional privilege: derived from the work of Dorothy Smith (1978), this refers broadly to the use by a teller of a story of the power to define what is true and untrue, normal or deviant.

Discourse: this may refer to language used within organizations or in encounters with service users, as this is displayed in talk, or written texts such as case notes. It may also refer to ways of thinking, or 'knowledges' or 'discourses' about particular phenomena, such as gender, race, the family or mental health, and how these reflect particular historical, political or moral positions.

Discourse analysis: a collection of research methods and analytical tools from diverse theoretical and disciplinary traditions. There is a preference for data that have 'naturally occurred' in the cut and thrust of everyday life. These are usually preserved on audiotape and transcribed using coding devices that attempt to represent as much of the detail of the interaction as possible. The context in which the talk takes place, or the audience for whom the accounts were written, is also of central importance. Analysts would be interested in the ways in which clinicians categorize and order their cases and how they use language strategically.

Discursive psychology: a branch of psychology concerned to remedy the neglect in traditional psychology of the subtleties of language use, and particularly its ambiguity and contestability. Discursive psychology draws on insights from *ethnomethodology, discourse, conversation, rhetoric* and *narrative analysis* and is particularly concerned with the capacity of language to 'perform' things in the world and to affect the ways in which individuals experience and think about it.

Enlightenment: a seventeenth-century philosophical movement that challenged traditional and religious ways of knowing, and was concerned with the pursuit of universal objective truth, and the separation of reason and emotion.

Epistemology: derived from the Greek *episteme*, meaning knowledge, to mean a theory of knowledge or ways of knowing with sets of associated ideas about validity and methods.

Ethnography: a collection of research methods originating in social anthropology and sociology that are used to understand people's daily lives and how these are shaped by interactions of various kinds. There are a number of different types of ethnography, e.g. analytic ethnography, critical ethnography and practitioner ethnography. However, these approaches all emphasize the ethnographer's 'deep familiarity' with the subjects studied. Analysis is built upon detailed descriptions of persons and events. Ethnographic research can expose aspects of professional practice that have become routine and unquestioned and thus has potential as a tool for the facilitation of *reflexive practice*.

Ethnomethodological ethnography: a type of ethnography concerned with how participants in a setting *constitute* reality through their activities – how they do things – within actual everyday situations (contrast with *interactionist ethnography*).

Ethnomethodology: derived originally from the work of Harold Garfinkel, this refers simply to 'folk' (ethno) 'methods' (ways of doing things). Ethnomethodology studies the complex forms of shared knowledge, upon which we all draw in making sense of and acting in everyday encounters with others.

Extreme case formulations: derived from the work of Pomerantz (1986), these are devices used in talk that invoke the maximal or minimal attributes of a person or event; for example, words like 'always', or 'never'. They are powerful devices for referencing blame (or creditworthiness) in talk.

Family systems theory: originates from general systems theory (von Bertalanffy 1971) which proposes that all organisms are systems, composed of sub-systems that are in turn part of super-systems. When applied to families, it posits that the problems of individual family members arise from patterns of relationships among family members and the family's interaction with wider social systems.

Foucauldian discourse analysis: derived from the work of philosopher, historian and social theorist Michel Foucault, this form of *discourse analysis* is concerned with how ideas come to affect the way we see and understand things and what effects these ideas have. Its focus is on 'knowledges' or 'discourses' about particular phenomena, such as gender, race, the family or mental health, and how these reflect particular historical, political or moral positions.

Hypothetico-deductive method: a scientific method derived from the work of Karl Popper (1959), which stresses the importance of falsification in testing the validity of a hypothesis. Competing hypotheses are successively 'falsified', through a rigorous search for disconfirming evidence, so that the hypothesis with the 'best fit' will prove most robust.

Indifferent kinds: these are ideas we have about objects, which have no capacity to answer back. Usually these will be part of the physical world, such as metals, gravity, blood or bone. They can act in various ways but they do so without consciousness. So, if a microbe makes us ill, it interacts with our bodies, but it does not know that it is doing so (contrast with *interactive kinds*).

Induction/inductive reasoning: a commitment to the production of new concepts from a position of openness. Theory emerges from observation and/or analysis of data, not the other way round (contrast with *deduction/ deductive reasoning*).

Interactionist ethnography: an ethnographic study concerned with the meanings actors in a setting ascribe to their practices (contrast with *ethnomethodological ethnography*).

Interactive kinds: this term derives from the work of Ian Hacking (1999) and refers to ideas, usually about people, that can, in some way, loop back into our ideas about ourselves and influence the ways we think and feel. Examples would include the ideas we have about childhood or being female, or about mental health and illness (contrast with *indifferent kinds*).

Interest or stake: The dilemma of stake or interest if exposed weakens the rhetorical effect of any account or argument. Thus, accounts that appear to be simple, not interpreted and unmotivated descriptions carry greater rhetorical effect.

Judgement analysis: is derived ecological psychology and posits that judgements are always mediated by various situational 'cues'. These processes can be represented as statistical formulae. It examines clinicians' judgement-making 'policy' and then creates a statistical representation of that 'policy'. These statistical representations are also used to generate predictions allegedly more accurate than the judges' own unassisted predictions.

Membership categorization: Membership categories are used in talk and text to assign individuals to social categories such as 'woman', 'mother', 'father', 'child', 'nurse', 'doctor'. These categorizations are linked to certain expectable behaviours or *category bound activities*, which may be breached. For example, if the category bound expectations of a person in the category 'mother' are that she will be nurturing and caring, a description of behaviour deviating from this expectation will mark deviance.

Membership categorization devices: these are collections of membership categories, such as 'family', which includes categories like mother, child, father, or 'occupation', which may include 'doctor', 'social worker', 'nurse'.

Modernity: refers to the 'age of reason', which is generally traced to the *Enlightenment* in Western Europe. The key themes of modernity are reason and progress.

Minimal response tokens: short verbal or non-verbal utterances in conversation (for example, Mm, Ehm), which can signal assent or dissent and invite the speaker to carry on speaking.

Narrative: usually defined as a particular kind of 'recapitulation', which presents events as the antecedents or consequences of each other. These kinds of consequential accounts attribute cause and effect in particular ways. Narratives can be analysed for their structural features, their characterizations and their effects. Professional work depends to a large extent on storytelling and narrative.

Nosologies: diagnostic categories and classifications of disease associated with biomedicine.

Realism: a philosophical position which claims that truths about the world exist independently of the 'knower'. The point of inquiry is to find out facts that remain the same no matter how we describe them.

Relativism: a philosophical position that disputes the realist stance that we can produce ultimate, universal truths about the world, which will correspond with independent reality. Relativism does not dispute the existence of an outside world but instead questions our unmediated access to it. Truth is therefore more provisional and subject to change and debate.

Rhetoric/rhetorical: in this book we use this term to refer to powerful and potent words and phrases deployed in talk and text. Rhetoric is not a contrast to factual reporting. Instead, it mobilizes facts in certain ways to achieve particular effects.

Rhetoric of deliberate vagueness: deliberate or systematic vagueness is a rhetorical device that can protect the speaker against easy undermining or rebuttal, while at the same time 'providing just the essentials to found a particular inference' (Edwards and Potter 1992: 162).

Social constructionism: an *epistemological* position which asserts that our ideas about the world do not straightforwardly describe it; instead, our language and ways of thinking 'construct' the world in particular ways (compare with *relativism*).

Standardized relational pairs: these are *membership categories* that often occur in pairs such as mother/child and that set up expectable sets of relationships between the parts of the pair.

Tacit knowledge: derived from the work of Polanyi (1967), and refers to taken-for-granted knowledge that allows us to perform certain activities without consciously thinking about them.

Vade mecum: derives from Latin and literally translated means 'go with me'. In English, vade mecum means a handbook or other reference aid. It is simplified takeaway knowledge – 'knowledge to go'.

Recommended further reading

We provide here a brief list of reading pertaining to the various topics discussed. The references are grouped by topic area, but it should be noted that many belong to more than one category. The following text, which applies discourse analysis to professional practice, should be considered a companion volume to this book:

Taylor, C. and White, S. (2000) *Practising Reflexivity in Health and Welfare: Making Knowledge*. Buckingham: Open University Press.

Clinical judgement

There is a vast literature on clinical judgement, much of which originates in psychology. For a detailed introduction to the various approaches see:

Dowie, J. and Elstein, A. (eds) (1988) *Professional Judgement: A Reader in Clinical Decision Making*. Cambridge: Cambridge University Press.

The following text includes useful chapters on a range of specific occupations, such as physiotherapy:

Higgs, J. and Jones, M. (eds) (2000) *Clinical Reasoning in the Health Professions*. Oxford: Butterworth Heinemann.

For a more detailed discussion of the concept of humane judgement we recommend:

Downie, R. S. and Macnaughton, J. (2000) *Clinical Judgement: Evidence in Practice*. Oxford: Oxford University Press.
Little, M. (1995) *Humane Medicine*. Cambridge: Cambridge University Press.

Qualitative research

Silverman, D. (1993) *Interpreting Qualitative Data: Methods for Analysing Talk, Text and Interaction*. London: Sage.
Silverman, D. (2000) *Doing Qualitative Research: A Practical Handbook*. London: Sage.
Coffey, A. and Atkinson, P. (1996) *Making Sense of Qualitative Data*. London: Sage.

David Silverman has written a number of accessible but rigorous texts on qualitative research. His own empirical work is in medical sociology, which means that many of his examples are drawn from health and welfare contexts. Any of his numerous books will provide useful guidance on methods for analysing talk, text and interaction. They include examples and exercises to help with the application of knowledge.

For those interested specifically in ethnography the following guide is a very well respected introduction. However, you should also try to read some empirical studies relevant to your area of work (see below):

Hammersley, M. and Atkinson, P. (1995) *Ethnography: Principles in Practice*, 2nd edn. London: Routledge.

Social constructionism and professional practice

If this material is unfamiliar, it may help to start by looking at a textbook that sets out the main perspectives within the social sciences, with specific sections on symbolic interactionism, ethnomethodology and Foucault. David Silverman's research guides provide this in an applied form, but you may also wish to try:

May, T. (1996) *Situating Social Theory*. Buckingham: Open University Press.

For a more specific analysis of social constructionism as applied to various phenomena, like child abuse or mental illness, see:

Hacking, I. (1999) *The Social Construction of What?* London: Harvard University Press.

Discursive psychology

We recommend the following to those who want to know more about the respecification of psychology:

Edwards, D. (1997) *Discourse and Cognition*. London: Sage.

Potter, J. (1996) *Representing Reality: Discourse, Rhetoric and Social Construction*. London: Sage.
Shotter, J. (1993) *Conversational Realities: Constructing Life through Language*. London: Sage.

Studies of talk and text in health and welfare

Collected works

Boden, D. and Zimmerman, D.H. (eds) (1991) *Talk and Social Structure: Studies in Ethnomethodology and Conversation Analysis*. Cambridge: Polity Press.
Drew, P. and Heritage, J. (eds) (1992) *Talk at Work: Interaction in Institutional Settings*. Cambridge: Cambridge University Press.
Sarangi, S. and Roberts, C. (1999) *Talk, Work and Institutional Order: Discourse in Medical, Mediation and Management Settings*. Berlin: Mouton de Gruyter.

Social workers

Hall, C. (1997) *Social Work as Narrative: Story Telling and Persuasion in Professional Texts*. Aldershot: Ashgate.

Doctors

Atkinson, P. (1995) *Medical Talk and Medical Work*. London: Sage.
Silverman, D. (1987) *Communication and Medical Practice*. London: Sage.
Strong, P. (1979) *The Ceremonial Order of the Clinic*. London: Routledge and Kegan Paul.

Nurses

Latimer, J. (2000) *The Conduct of Care: Understanding Nursing Practice*. Oxford: Blackwell Science.
Wicks, D. (1998) *Nurses and Doctors at Work: Rethinking Professional Boundaries*. Buckingham: Open University Press.

Health visitors

Heritage, J. and Sefi, S. (1992) Dilemmas of advice: aspects of the delivery and reception of advice in interactions between health visitors and first-time mothers. In P. Drew and J. Heritage (eds) *Talk at Work: Interaction in Institutional Settings*. Cambridge: Cambridge University Press.

Family therapy

Buttny, R. and Jensen, A. D. (1995) Telling problems in an initial family therapy session: the hierarchical organisation of problem-talk. In G. H. Morris and R. J. Chenail (eds) *The Talk of the Clinic: Explorations of Medical and Therapeutic Discourse*. Hillsdale, NJ: Lawrence Erlbaum.

Gubrium, J. F. (1992) *Out of Control: Family Therapy and Domestic Disorder*. Newbury Park, CA: Sage.

Miller, G. (1987) Producing family problems: organization and uses of the family perspective and rhetoric in family therapy. *Symbolic Interaction*, 10(2), 245–65.

Counselling

Miller, G. and Silverman, D. (1995) Troubles talk and counselling discourse: a comparative study. *Sociological Quarterly*, 36(4), 725–47.

Peräkylä, A. (1995) *AIDS Counselling: Institutional Interaction and Clinical Practice*. Cambridge: Cambridge University Press.

Silverman, D. (1997) *Discourses of Counselling: HIV Counselling as Social Interaction*. London: Sage.

Social studies of science

Many of the texts in this area are quite dense and not very accessible to those unfamiliar with the concepts. However, for those with a specific interest, it is well worth persevering – it does get easier!

Fleck, L. (1979) *Genesis and Development of Scientific Fact*. Chicago: University of Chicago Press.

Latour, B. (1999) *Pandora's Hope: Essays on the Reality of Science Studies*. London: Harvard University Press.

Latour, B. and Woolgar, S. (1986) *Laboratory Life: The Construction of Scientific Facts*. Princeton, NJ: Princeton University Press.

Law J. (ed.) (1991) *A Sociology of Monsters*. London: Routledge.

Law, J. (1994) *Organizing Modernity*. Oxford: Blackwell.

Lynch, M. and Woolgar, S. (eds) (1990) *Representation in Scientific Practice*. Cambridge, MA: MIT Press.

Thagard, P. (2000) *How Scientists Explain Disease*. Princeton, NJ: Princeton University Press.

Emotion and reasoning

Damasio, A. R. (1994) *Descartes' Error: Emotion, Reason and the Human Brain*l. New York: Avon Books.

Damasio, A. (1999) *The Feeling of What Happens: Body, Emotion and the Making of Consciousness*. London: Heinemann.

De Sousa, R. (1991) *The Rationality of Emotion*. Cambridge, MA: MIT Press.

References

Anderson, H. and Goolishian, H. A. (1992) The client is the expert: a not-knowing approach to therapy. In S. McNamee and K. J. Gergen (eds) *Therapy as a Social Construction*. London: Sage.

Anspach, R. (1987) Prognostic conflict in life-and-death decisions: the organization as an ecology of knowledge. *Journal of Health and Social Behaviour*, 28(3), 215–31.

Anspach, R. (1988) Notes on the sociology of medical discourse: the language of case presentation. *Journal of Health and Social Behaviour*, 29, 357–75.

Atkinson, P. (1990) *The Ethnographic Imagination*. London: Routledge.

Atkinson, P. (1995) *Medical Talk and Medical Work*. London: Sage.

Aull Davies, C. (1999) *Reflexive Ethnography: A Guide to Researching Selves and Others*. London: Routledge.

Baker, T. (1995) What constitutes reasonable contact? In P. Reder and C. Lucey (eds) *Assessment of Parenting: Psychiatric and Psychological Contributions*. London: Routledge.

Bateson, G. (1978) *Steps to an Ecology of Mind: Collected Essays in Anthropology, Psychiatry, Evolution and Epistemology*. London: Paladin/Granada Publishing.

Benner, P. (1984) *From Novice to Expert: Excellence and Power in Clinical Nursing Practice*. Menlo Park, CA: Addison-Wesley.

Benner, P., Tanner, C. A. and Chesla, C. A. (1996) *Expertise in Nursing Practice: Caring, Clinical Judgement and Ethics*. New York: Springer.

Berg, M. (1997) *Rationalizing Medical Work: Decision Support Techniques and Medical Practices*. Cambridge, MA: MIT Press.

Billig, M. (ed.) (1991) *Ideology and Opinions: Studies in Rhetorical Psychology*. London: Sage.

Billig, M., Condor, S., Edwards, D., Grane, M., Middleton, D. and Radley A. (1988) *Ideological Dilemmas: A Social Psychology of Everyday Thinking*. London: Sage.

Bloor, M. (1976) Bishop Berkeley and the adeno-tonsillectomy enigma: an exploration of variation in the social construction of medical disposal. *Sociology*, 10, 43–61.

Bloor, M. (1994) On the conceptualisation of routine decision-making: death certification as an habitual activity. In M. Bloor and P. Tarborelli (eds) *Qualitative Studies in Health and Medicine*. Cardiff Papers in Qualitative Research. Aldershot: Avebury.

Bloor, M. (1997) Addressing social problems through qualitative research. In D. Silverman (ed.) *Qualitative Research: Theory, Method, Practice*. London: Sage.

Boden, D. and Zimmerman, D. H. (eds) (1991) *Talk and Social Structure: Studies in Ethnomethodology and Conversation Analysis*. Cambridge: Polity Press.

Boscolo, L., Checchin, G., Hoffman, L. and Penn, P. (1987) Training in systemic therapy at the Milan Centre. In R. Whiffen and J. Byng-Hall (eds) *Family Therapy Supervision: Recent Developments in Practice*. London: Academic Press.

Bosk, C. L. (1979) *Forgive and Remember: Managing Medical Failure*. Chicago: University of Chicago Press.

Bowlby, J. and Salter-Ainsworth, M. (1969) *Child Care and the Growth of Love*, 2nd edn. Harmondsworth: Penguin.

Bradbury, M. (1999) *Representations of Death: A Social Psychological Perspective*. London: Routledge.

Brewer, J. (1994) The ethnographic critique of ethnography. *Sociology*, 28(1), 231–44.

Brooks, L. R., Norman, G. R. and Allen, S. W. (1991) Role of specific similarity in a medical diagnostic task. *Journal of Experimental Psychology, General*, 120, 278–87.

Brown, P. and Levinson, S. C. (1987) *Politeness: Some Universals in Language Usage*. Cambridge: Cambridge University Press.

Bryant, C. G. A. (1991) The dialogical model of applied sociology. In C. G. A. Bryant and D. Jary (eds) *Giddens' Theory of Structuration: A Critical Appreciation*. London: Routledge.

Burman, E. (1990) Time, language and power in modern developmental psychology. Unpublished PhD thesis, University of Manchester.

Burman, E. (1994) *Deconstructing Developmental Psychology*. London: Routledge.

Butler-Sloss, E. (1988) *Report of the Inquiry into Child Abuse in Cleveland*. London: HMSO.

Buttny, R. (1993) *Social Accountability in Communication*. London: Sage.

Buttny, R. and Jensen, A. D. (1995) Telling problems in an initial family therapy session: the hierarchical organisation of problem-talk. In G. H. Morris and R. J. Chenail (eds) *The Talk of the Clinic: Explorations of Medical and Therapeutic Discourse*. Hillsdale, NJ: Lawrence Erlbaum.

Canadian Task Force on the Periodic Health Examination (1979) Taskforce report: the periodic health examination. *Canadian Medical Journal*, 314, 1118–22.

Cicourel, A. (1999) The interaction of cognitive and cultural models in health care delivery. In S. Sarangi and C. Roberts (eds) *Talk, Work and Institutional Order: Discourse in Medical, Mediation and Management Settings*. Berlin: Mouton de Gruyter.

Clarke, A. (1991) Is non-directive genetic counselling possible? *The Lancet*, 338, 998–1001.

Clavarino, A., Najman, J. and Silverman, D. (1995) Assessing the quality of qualitative data. *Qualitative Inquiry*, 1(2), 223–42.

Clayman, S. (1988) Displaying neutrality in news interviews. *Social Problems*, 35(4), 474–92.

Code, L. (1995) *Rhetorical Spaces: Essays on Gendered Locations*. New York: Routledge.

Coffey, A. and Atkinson, P. (1996) *Making Sense of Qualitative Data*. London: Sage.

Cooksey, R. W. (1996) *Judgement Analysis: Theory, Method and Applications*. San Diego: Academic Press.

Cuff, E. (1993) *Problems of Versions in Everyday Situations*. Lanham, MD: University Press of America.

Dahlberg, G., Moss, P. and Pence, A. (1999) *Beyond Quality in Early Childhood Education and Care: Postmodern Perspectives*. London: Falmer Press.

Daly, J. (1989) Innocent murmurs: echocardiography and the diagnosis of cardiac abnormality. *Sociology of Health and Illness*, 11, 99–116.

Damasio, A. R. (1994) *Descartes' Error: Emotion, Reason and the Human Brain*. New York: Avon Books.

Damasio, A. (1999) *The Feeling of What Happens: Body, Emotion and the Making of Consciousness*. London: Heinemann.

Davidoff, F. (1998) Is basic science necessary? In F. Davidoff, *Who Has Seen a Blood Sugar? Reflections on Medical Education*. Philadelphia: American College of Physicians.

de Dombal, F. T. (1989) Computer-aided decision support in clinical medicine. *International Journal of Biomedicine and Computing*, 24, 9–16.

de Dombal F. T., Leaper, D. J., Staniland, J. R., McCann, A. P. and Horrocks, J. C. (1972) Computer-aided diagnosis of acute abdominal pain. *British Medical Journal*, 302, 1495–7.

Delamont, S. and Atkinson, P. (2001) Doctoring uncertainty: mastering craft knowledge. *Social Studies of Science*, 31(1), 87–107.

Department of Health (1997) *The New NHS Modern, Dependable*. London: The Stationery Office.

Department of Health (2001a) New social care institute for excellence will raise standards and tackle inconsistencies. Press release 0100, 25 February (http://www.childrenuk.co.uk/chmay2001/news/soc%20care%20institute%20doh.htm).

Department of Health (2001b) Treatment choice in psychological therapies and counselling: evidence based clinical practice guideline (http://www.doh.gov.uk/mentalhealth/treatmentguideline/).

De Sousa, R. (1991) *The Rationality of Emotion*. Cambridge, MA: MIT Press.

Dingwall, R. (1977) 'Atrocity stories' and professional relationships. *Sociology of Work and Occupations*, 4(4), 371–96.

Dingwall, R. and Murray, T. (1983) Categorisation in accident departments: 'good' patients, 'bad' patients and 'children'. *Sociology of Health and Illness*, 5(2), 127–48.

Dowie, J. and Elstein, A. (eds) (1988) *Professional Judgement: A Reader in Clinical Decision Making*. Cambridge: Cambridge University Press.

Downie, R. S. and Charlton, B. (1992) *The Making of a Doctor: Medical Education in Theory and Practice*. Oxford: Oxford University Press.

Downie, R. S. and Macnaughton, J. (2000) *Clinical Judgement: Evidence in Practice.* Oxford: Oxford University Press.

Drew, P. and Heritage, J. (eds) (1992) *Talk at Work: Interaction in Institutional Settings.* Cambridge: Cambridge University Press.

Eddy, D. M. (1988) Variations in physician practice: the role of uncertainty. In J. Dowie and A. Elstein (eds) *Professional Judgement: A Reader in Clinical Decision Making.* Cambridge: Cambridge University Press.

Edwards, D. (1997) *Discourse and Cognition.* London: Sage.

Edwards, D., Ashmore, M. and Potter, J. (1995) Death and furniture: the rhetoric, politics and theology of bottom line arguments against relativism. *History of the Human Sciences*, 8(2), 25–49.

Edwards, D. and Potter, J. (1992) *Discursive Psychology.* London: Sage.

Einhorn, H. J. (1988) Accepting more error to make less error. In J. Dowie and A. Elstein (eds) *Professional Judgement: A Reader in Clinical Decision Making.* Cambridge: Cambridge University Press.

Elliott, R. and Anderson, C. (1994) Simplicity and complexity in psychotherapy research. In R. L. Russell (ed.) *Reassessing Psychotherapy Research.* New York: Guilford Press.

Elstein, A. S. (1994) What goes around comes around: the return of the hypothetico-deductive strategy. *Teaching and Learning in Medicine*, 6, 121–3.

Elstein, A. S. and Schwartz, A. (2000) Clinical reasoning in medicine. In J. Higgs and M. Jones (eds) *Clinical Reasoning in the Health Professions.* Oxford: Butterworth Heinemann.

Elwyn, G., Gray, J. and Clarke, A. (2000) Shared decision-making and non-directiveness in genetic counselling. *Journal of Medical Genetics*, 37, 135–8.

Elwyn, G. and Gwyn, R. (1999) Stories we hear and stories we tell: analysing talk in clinical practice. *British Medical Journal*, 318, 186–8.

Epstein, E. (1993) From irreverence to irrelevance? The growing disjuncture of family therapy theories from social realities. *Journal of Systemic Therapies*, 12(3), 15–27.

Epstein, E. and Loos, V. E. (1989) Some irreverent thoughts on the limits of family therapy. *Journal of Family Psychology*, 2(4), 405–21.

Eraut, M. (1994) *Developing Professional Knowledge and Competence.* London: Falmer Press.

Eva, K. W., Neville, A. J. and Norman, G. R. (1998) Exploring the etiology of content specificity: factors influencing analogic transfer and problem solving. *Academic Medicine*, 73, S1–S5.

Fahlberg, V. (1979) *Attachment and Separation.* London: British Agencies for Adoption and Fostering.

Feinstein, A. R. (1977) Clinical biostatistics xxxix: the haze of Bayes, the aerial palaces of decision analysis and the computerized Ouija board. *Clinical Pharmacology and Therapeutics*, 21, 482–96.

Fischhoff, B. and Beyth-Marom, R. (1988) Hypothesis evaluation from a Bayesian perspective. In J. Dowie and A. Elstein (eds) *Professional Judgement: A Reader in Clinical Decision Making*. Cambridge: Cambridge University Press.

Fleck, L. (1979) *Genesis and Development of Scientific Fact*. Chicago: University of Chicago Press.

Flynn, R. (1992) *Structures of Control in Health Service Management*. London: Routledge.

Flynn, R. and Williams, G. (eds) (1997) *Contracting for Health*. Oxford: Oxford University Press.

Foucault, M. (1973) *The Birth of the Clinic: An Archaeology of Medical Perception*. New York: Vintage Books.

Foucault, M. (1976) *Mental Illness and Psychology*. New York: Harper Colophon.

Foucault, M. (1980) *Power/Knowledge: Selected Interviews and Other Writings 1972–1977* (ed. C. Gordon). Hemel Hempstead: Harvester Wheatsheaf.

Foucault, M. (1994) An interview with Simon Riggins. In P. Rabinow (ed.) *Michel Foucault. Ethics: The Essential Works*. London: Penguin.

Frosh, S. (1991) The semantics of therapeutic change. *Journal of Family Therapy*, 13, 171–86.

Frosh, S. (1997) *For and Against Psychoanalysis*. London: Routledge.

Garfinkel, H. (1967) *Studies in Ethnomethodology*. Cambridge: Polity Press.

Garfinkel, H. and Sacks, H. (1970) On formal structures of practical actions. In J. C. McKinney and E. Tirakian (eds) *Theoretical Sociology*. New York: Appleton Century Crofts.

Garralda, M. E. (1994) Chronic physical illness and emotional disorder in childhood. *British Journal of Psychiatry*, 164, 8–10.

Garralda, M. E. (1996) Somatisation in children. *Journal of Child Psychology, Psychiatry and Allied Disciplines*, 37(1), 13–33.

Geertz, C. (1973) *The Interpretation of Cultures: Selected Essays*. New York: Basic Books.

Geertz, C. (1979) From the native's point of view: on the nature of anthropological understanding. In P. Rabinow and W. M. Sullivan (eds) *Interpretive Social Science: A Reader*. Berkeley: University of California Press.

Giddens, A. (1987) *Social Theory and Modern Sociology*. Cambridge: Polity Press.

Glaser, B. and Strauss, A. (1965) *Awareness of Dying*. Chicago: Aldine.

Glaser, B. and Strauss, A. (1968) *A Time for Dying*. Chicago: Aldine.

Goffman, E. (1959) *The Presentation of Self in Everyday Life*. New York: Doubleday.

Goffman, E. (1961) *Asylums*. New York: Doubleday.

Goffman, E. (1967) *Interaction Ritual: Essays on Face to Face Behaviour*. Garden City, NY: Doubleday Anchor.

Golann, S. (1988) On second order family therapy. *Family Process*, 27, 51–65.

Goldberg, L. R. (1970) Man versus model of man: a rationale, plus some evidence for a method of improving on clinical inferences. *Psychological Bulletin*, 73, 422–32.

Goldner, V. (1991) Feminism and systemic practice: two critical traditions in transition. *Journal of Family Therapy*, 13, 95–104.

Gomm, R. (2000) Making sense of surveys. In R. Gomm and C. Davies (eds) *Using Evidence in Health and Social Care*. London: Sage.

Graham, I. (1998) Understanding the nature of nursing through reflection: a case study approach. In C. Johns and D. Freshwater (eds) *Transforming Nursing through Reflective Practice*. Oxford: Blackwell.

Greatbatch, D. and Dingwall, R. (1999) Professional neutralism in family mediation. In S. Sarangi and C. Roberts (eds) *Talk, Work and Institutional Order: Discourse in Medical, Mediation and Management Settings*. Berlin: Mouton de Gruyter.

Green, J. (2000) Epistemology, evidence and experience: evidence based health care in the work of Accident Alliances. *Sociology of Health and Illness*, 22(4), 453–76.

Greenhalgh, T. (1999) Narrative based medicine in an evidence based world. *British Medical Journal*, 318, 323–5.

Greenhalgh, T. and Hurwitz, B. (1999) Narrative based medicine: why study narrative? *British Medical Journal*, 318, 48–50.

Groen, G. J. and Patel, V. L. (1985) Medical problem solving: some questionable assumptions. *Medical Education*, 19, 95–100.

Grosskurth, P. (1986) *Melanie Klein: Her World and Her Work*. London: Maresfield Books.

Gubrium, J. F. (1992) *Out of Control: Family Therapy and Domestic Disorder*. Newbury Park, CA: Sage.

Hacking, I. (1999) *The Social Construction of What?* London: Harvard University Press.

Hall, C. (1997) *Social Work as Narrative: Storytelling and Persuasion in Professional Texts*. Aldershot: Ashgate.

Hall, C. and Slembrook, S. (2002) Caring-but-not-coping: fashioning a legitimate parent identity. In C. Hall, K. Juhila, N. Parton and T. Poso (eds) *Constructing Clienthood in Social Work and Human Services*. London: Jessica Kingsley.

Hall, S. (1992) Cultural studies and its theoretical legacies. In L. Grossberg, C. Nelso and P. Treichler (eds) *Cultural Studies*. London: Routledge.

Ham, C. (1999) *Health Policy in Britain: The Politics and Organisation of the National Health Service*. Basingstoke: Macmillan.

Hammersley, M. (1992) *What's Wrong with Ethnography?* London: Routledge.

Hammersley, M. and Atkinson, P. (1995) *Ethnography: Principles in Practice*, 2nd edn. London: Routledge.

Hargreaves, A. (1981) Contrastive rhetoric and extremist talk: teachers, hegemony and the educationalist context. In L. Barton and S. Walker (eds) *Schools, Teachers and Teaching*. Lewes: Falmer Press.

Harrison, S. (1998) The politics of evidence-based medicine in the United Kingdom. *Policy and Politics*, 26(1), 15–31.

Harrison, S. (1999) New Labour, modernisation and health care governance. Paper presented at the Political Studies Association/Social Policy Association conference 'New Labour, New Health', London, September.

Harrison, S. and Ahmed, W. I. (2000) Medical autonomy and the UK state 1975–2025. *Sociology*, 34(1), 129–46.

Harrison, S. and Pollitt, C. (1994) *Controlling Health Professionals: The Future of Work and Organization in the NHS*. Buckingham: Open University Press.

Herbert, M. (1996) Assessing children in need and their parents. In *The PACTS Series: Parent, Adolescent and Child Training Skills*. Leicester: BPS Books.

Heritage, J. and Sefi, S. (1992) Dilemmas of advice: aspects of the delivery and reception of advice in interactions between health visitors and first-time mothers. In P. Drew and J. Heritage (eds) *Talk at Work: Interaction in Institutional Settings*. Cambridge: Cambridge University Press.

Higgs, J. and Jones, M. (eds) (200) *Clinical Reasoning in the Health Professions*. Oxford: Butterworth Heinemann.

Hollon, S. D. (1996) The efficacy and effectiveness of psychotherapy relative to medications. *American Psychologist*, 51(10), 1025–30.

Hollway, W. and Jefferson, T. (2000) *Doing Qualitative Research Differently: Free Association, Narrative and the Interview Method*. London: Sage.

Housley, W. (2000) Category work and knowledgeability within multidisciplinary team meetings. *TEXT*, 20(1), 83–107.

Housley, W. and Fitzgerald, R (2002) The reconsidered model of membership categorization analysis. *Qualitative Research*, 2(1), 59–83.

Hunter, K. M. (1991) *Doctors' Stories: The Narrative Structure of Medical Knowledge*. Princeton, NJ: Princeton University Press.

Ivey, D. C., Scheel, M. and Jankowski, P. J. (1999) A contextual perspective of clinical judgement in couples and family therapy: is the bridge too far? *Journal of Family Therapy*, 21, 339–59.

Ixer, G. (1999) There is no such thing as reflection. *British Journal of Social Work*, 29(4), 513–28.

Jayussi, L. (1984) *Categorization and the Moral Order*. London: Routledge.

Jayussi, L. (1991) Values and moral judgement. In *Ethnomethodology and the Human Sciences*. Cambridge: Cambridge University Press.

Jeffrey, R. (1979) Normal rubbish: deviant patients in casualty departments. *Sociology of Health and Illness*, 1, 90–107.

John, I. D. (1990) Discursive style and psychological practice. *Australian Psychologist*, 25(2), 115–32.

Kahneman, D., Sloveic, P. and Tversky, A. (1982) *Judgement Under Uncertainty: Heuristics and Biases*. New York: Cambridge University Press.

Kaye, J. (1995) Postfoundationalism and the language of psychotherapy research. In J. Siegfried (ed.) *The Status of Common Sense in Psychology*. New York: Ablex.

Kessler, S. (1997) Psychological aspects of genetic counseling, XI. Nondirectiveness revisited. *American Journal of Medical Genetics*, 72, 164–71.

Kiesler, D. J. (1966) Some myths of psychotherapy research and the search for a paradigm. *Psychological Bulletin*, 65, 110–36.

Knorr-Cetina, K. and Mulkay, M. (1983) Introduction: emerging principles in the social study of science. In K. Knorr-Cetina and M. Mulkay (eds) *Science Observed: Perspectives on the Social Study of Science*. Beverley Hills, CA: Sage.

Kuhn, T. (1970) *The Structure of Scientific Revolutions*. Chicago: Chicago University Press.

Kuhn, T. (1993) Afterwords. In P. Horwich (ed.) *World Changes: Thomas Kuhn and the Nature of Science*. Cambridge, MA: MIT Press.

Lannamann, J. W. (1989) Communication theory applied to relational change: a case study in Milan systems family therapy. *Journal of Applied Communication Research*, 17, 71–91.

Latimer, J. (2000) *The Conduct of Care: Understanding Nursing Practice*. Oxford: Blackwell Science.

Latour, B. (1999) *Pandora's Hope: Essays on the Reality of Science Studies*. London: Harvard University Press.

Latour, B. and Woolgar, S. (1986) *Laboratory Life: The Construction of Scientific Facts*. Princeton, NJ: Princeton University Press.

Launer, J. (1999) A narrative approach to mental health in general practice. *British Medical Journal*, 318, 117–19.

Launer, J. (2001) Whatever happened to biology? Reconnecting family therapy with its evolutionary origins. *Journal of Family Therapy*, 23(2), 155–70.

Law, J. (ed.) (1991) *A Sociology of Monsters*. London: Routledge.

Law, J. (1994) *Organizing Modernity*. Oxford: Blackwell.

Little, M. (1995) *Humane Medicine*. Cambridge: Cambridge University Press.

Lloyd, R. M. (1992) Negotiating child sexual abuse: the interactional character of investigative practices. *Social Problems*, 39(2), 109–24.

Lynch, M. and Woolgar, S. (eds) (1990) *Representation in Scientific Practice*. Cambridge, MA: MIT Press.

Macdonald, G. (1994) Developing empirically-based practice in probation. *British Journal of Social Work*, 24, 405–27.

Macdonald, G. (1998) Promoting evidence-based practice in child protection. *Clinical Child Psychology and Psychiatry*, 3(1), 71–85.

McHugh, P. (1970) A common-sense conception of deviance. In J. D. Douglas (ed.) *Deviance and Respectability: The Social Construction of Moral Meaning*. New York: Basic Books.

McNeish, D., Newman, T. and Roberts, H. (2002) *What Works for Children?* Buckingham: Open University Press.

Malinowski, B. (1922) *Argonauts of the Western Pacific*. London: Routledge.

Marks, D. (1993) Case-conference analysis and action research. In E. Burman and I. Parker (eds) *Discourse Analytic Research: Repertoires and Readings of Texts in Action*. London: Routledge.

Marks, D. (1995) Gendered 'care' and the structuring of group relations:

child–professional–parent–researcher. In E. Burman, P. Aldred, C. Bewley, B. Goldberg, C. Heenan, D. Marks, J. Marshall, K. Taylor, R. Ullah and S. Warner, *Challenging Women: Psychology's Exclusions, Feminist Possibilities*. Buckingham: Open University Press.

May, C. (1992a) Individual care: power and subjectivity in therapeutic relationships. *Sociology*, 26, 589–602.

May, C. (1992b) Nursing work, nurses' knowledge and the subjectification of the patient. *Sociology of Health and Illness*, 14, 472–87.

May, T. (1996) *Situating Social Theory*. Buckingham: Open University Press.

Maynard, D. (1989) On the ethnography and analysis of discourse in institutional settings. *Perspectives on Social Problems*, 1, 127–46.

Meadow, R. (1980) Factitious epilepsy. *Lancet*, 1, 25.

Meadow, R. (1985) Management of Munchausen syndrome by proxy. *Archives of Disease in Childhood*, 60, 385.

Miller, G. and Silverman, D. (1995) Troubles talk and counselling discourse: a comparative study. *Sociological Quarterly*, 36(4), 725–47.

Mishler, E. G. (1986) *Research Interviewing: Context and Narrative*. Cambridge: Cambridge University Press.

Mitchell, J. C. (1983) Case and situational analysis. *Sociological Review*, 50(3), 273–88.

Mitchie, S., Bron, F., Bobrow, M. and Marteau, T. M. (1997) Nondirectiveness in genetic counselling: an empirical study. *American Journal of Human Genetics*, 60, 40–7.

Murphy, E., Dingwall, R., Greatbatch, D., Parker, S. and Watson, P. (1998) Qualitative research methods in health technology assessment: a review of the literature. *Health Technology Assessment*, 2 (complete part 16).

New, B. (1996) The rationing agenda in the NHS. *British Medical Journal*, 312, 1593–601.

NHS Executive (1998) *A First Class Service*. London: Department of Health.

Norman, G. R., Coblentz, C. L., Brooks, L. R. and Smith, E. K. M. (1994) Cognitive differences in clinical reasoning related to postgraduate training. *Teaching and Learning in Medicine*, 6, 114–20.

Orlinsky, D. E. and Howard K. I. (1994) Tradition and change in psychotherapy research: notes in the fourth generation. In R. Russell (ed.) *Reassessing Psychotherapy Research*. New York: Guilford Press.

Owen, I. R. (1999) The future of psychotherapy in the UK: discussing clinical governance. *British Journal of Psychotherapy*, 16(2), 197–207.

Parry, G. and Richardson, A. (1996) *NHS Psychotherapy Services in England: Review of Strategic Developments*. Wetherby: Department of Health.

Pasveer, B. (1989) Knowledge of shadows: the introduction of X-ray images in medicine. *Sociology of Health and Illness*, 11, 360–81.

Peräkylä, A. (1995) *AIDS Counselling: Institutional Interaction and Clinical Practice*. Cambridge: Cambridge University Press.

Peters, R. S. (1966) *Ethics and Education*. London: Routledge and Kegan Paul.

Piaget, J. (1958) *The Child's Construction of Reality*. London: Routledge and Kegan Paul.

Polanyi, M. (1967) *The Tacit Dimension*. London: Routledge and Kegan Paul.

Pomerantz, A. M. (1978) Attributions of responsibility: blamings. *Sociology*, 12, 115–21.

Pomerantz, A. M. (1986) Extreme case formulations: a new way of legitimating claims. *Human Studies*, 9, 219–30.

Popper, K. (1959) *The Logic of Scientific Discovery*. London: Hutchinson.

Popper, K. (1972) *Objective Knowledge*. Oxford: Clarendon Press.

Potter, J. (1982) 'Nothing so practical as a good theory'. The problematic application of social psychology. In P. Stringer (ed.) *Confronting Social Issues, Volume 1*. London: Academic Books.

Potter, J. (1996) *Representing Reality: Discourse, Rhetoric and Social Construction*. London: Sage.

Potter, J., Edwards, D. and Ashmore, M.(1999) Regulating criticism: some comments on an argumentative complex. *History of the Human Sciences*, 12(4), 79–88.

Potter, J. and Wetherell, M. (1995) Discourse analysis. In J. A. Smith, R. Harré and L. van Langrove (eds) *Rethinking Methods in Psychology*. London: Sage.

Reder, P. and Lucey, C. (eds) (1995) *Assessment of Parenting: Psychiatric and Psychological Contributions*. London: Routledge.

Reichardt, C. S. and Cook, T. D. (1979) Beyond qualitative versus quantitative methods. In T. D. Cook and C. S. Reichardt (eds) *Qualitative and Quantitative Methods in Evaluation Research*. Beverley Hills, CA: Sage.

Reiser, S. J. (1978) *Medicine and the Reign of Technology*. Cambridge: Cambridge University Press.

Reissman, C. K. (1993) *Narrative Analysis*. Newbury Park, CA: Sage.

Reissman, C. K. (2001) Personal troubles as social issues: a narrative of infertility in context. In I. Shaw and N. Gould (eds) *Qualitative Research in Social Work*. London: Sage.

Rolfe, G. (1998) *Expanding Nursing Knowledge: Understanding and Researching Your Own Practice*. Oxford: Butterworth Heinemann.

Rose, N. (1989) *Governing the Soul: The Shaping of the Private Self*. London: Routledge.

Rose, N. (1998) *Inventing Our Selves: Psychology, Power and Personhood*. Cambridge: Cambridge University Press.

Sackett, D. L., Richardson, S., Rosenberg, W. and Haynes, R. B. (1997) *Evidence-based Medicine: How to Practise and Teach EBM*. Edinburgh: Churchill-Livingstone.

Sacks, H. (1972) On the analyzability of stories by children. In J. Gumpertz and D. Hymes (eds) *Directions in Sociolinguistics: The Ethnography of Communication*. New York: Holt, Rinehart and Winston.

Sacks, H. (1992) *Lectures on Conversation* (ed. G. Jefferson). Oxford: Blackwell.

Sacks, H., Schegloff, E. A. and Jefferson, G. (1974) A simplest systematics for the organization of turn taking in conversation. *Language*, 50, 696–735.

Sarangi, S. and Roberts C. (eds) (1999) *Talk, Work and Institutional Order: Discourse in Medical, Mediation and Management Settings*. Berlin: Mouton de Gruyter.

Schön, D. A. (1983) *The Reflective Practitioner*. New York: Free Press.

Schön, D. A. (1987) *Educating the Reflective Practitioner: Towards a New Design for Teaching and Learning in the Professions*. San Francisco: Jossey-Bass.

Schön, D. A. (1988) From technical rationality to reflection-in-action. In J. Dowie and A. Elstein (eds) *Professional Judgement: A Reader in Clinical Decision Making*. Cambridge: Cambridge University Press.

Sechrest, L., McKnight, P. and McKnight, K. (1996) Calibration of measures for psychotherapy outcome studies. *American Psychologist*, 51(10), 1065–71.

Self, W. (1994) *The Quantity Theory of Insanity*. London: Penguin.

Seligman, M. E. P. (1996) Science as an ally of practice. *American Psychologist*, 51(10), 1072–9.

Sheldon, B. (1983) The use of single case experimental designs in the evaluation of social work effectiveness. *British Journal of Social Work*, 13, 3–17.

Sheldon, B. (1986) Social work effectiveness experiments: review and implications. *British Journal of Social Work*, 16, 223–42.

Sheldon, B. (1999) Cognitive behavioural methods in social care: a review of the evidence. In P. Stepney and D. Ford (eds) *Social Work Models, Methods and Theories: A Framework for Practice*. Lyme Regis: Russell House Publishing.

Sheldon, B. (2001) The validity of evidence-based practice in social work: a reply to Stephen Webb. *British Journal of Social Work*, 31, 801–9.

Sheldon, B. and MacDonald, G. M. (1999) *Research and Practice in Social Care: Mind the Gap*. Exeter: Centre for Evidence-Based Social Services, University of Exeter.

Sheppard, M. (1995) Social work, social science and practice wisdom. *British Journal of Social Work*, 25(3), 265–93.

Sheppard, M. (1998) Practice validity, reflexivity and knowledge. *British Journal of Social Work*, 28(5), 763–81.

Shotter, J. (1993) *Conversational Realities: Constructing Life through Language*. London: Sage.

Silverman, D. (1987) *Communication and Medical Practice*. London: Sage.

Silverman, D. (1993) *Interpreting Qualitative Data: Methods for Analysing Talk, Text and Interaction*. London: Sage.

Silverman, D. (ed.) (1997) *Qualitative Research: Theory, Method and Practice*. London: Sage.

Silverman, D. (1998) *Harvey Sacks: Social Science and Conversation Analysis*. Cambridge: Polity Press.

Silverman, D. (2000) *Doing Qualitative Research: A Practical Handbook*. London: Sage.

Silverman, D. and Gubrium, J. F. (1989) Introduction. In J. F. Gubrium and D. Silverman (eds) *The Politics of Field Research: Sociology Beyond the Enlightenment*. London: Sage.

Smith, D. (1978) K is mentally ill: the anatomy of a factual account. *Sociology*, 12, 23–53.

Snyder, M. and Thomsen, C. (1988) Interactions between therapists and clients: hypothesis testing and behavioural confirmation. In D. C. Turk and P. Salovey (eds) *Reasoning, Inference and Judgement in Clinical Psychology*. New York: Free Press.

Stainton Rogers, R. and Stainton Rogers, W. (1992) *Stories of Childhood: Shifting Agendas of Child Concern*. Hemel Hempstead: Harvester Wheatsheaf.

Stancombe, J. (2002) Family therapy as narrative: managing blame and responsibility. Unpublished PhD thesis, University of London.

Stancombe, J. and White, S. (1998) Psychotherapy without foundations: hermeneutics, discourse and the end of certainty. *Theory and Psychology*, 8(5), 579–99.

Stanley, L. (ed.) (1990) *Feminist Praxis: Research Theory and Epistemology in Feminist Sociology*. London: Routledge.

Stevenson, O. and Parsloe, P. (1978) *Social Services Teams: The Practitioners' View*. London: HMSO.

Stiles, W. B. (1988) Psychotherapy process-outcome correlations may be misleading. *Psychotherapy*, 25, 27–35.

Stiles, W. B. and Shapiro, D. A. (1989) Abuse of the drug metaphor in psychotherapy process-outcome research. *Clinical Psychology Review*, 9, 521–43.

Stiles, W. B., Shapiro, D. A. and Elliott, R. (1986) Are all psychotherapies equivalent? *American Psychologist*, 41, 165–80.

Stiles, W. B., Shapiro, D. A. and Harper, H. (1994) Finding the ways from process to outcome: blind alleys and unmarked trails. In R. Russell (ed.) *Reassessing Psychotherapy Research*. New York: Guilford Press.

Strong, P. (1979) *The Ceremonial Order of the Clinic*. London: Routledge and Kegan Paul.

Sudnow, D. (1968) *Passing On: The Social Organization of Dying*. Englewood Cliffs, NJ: Prentice Hall.

Taylor, C. and White, S. (2000) *Practising Reflexivity in Health and Welfare: Making Knowledge*. Buckingham: Open University Press.

Taylor, C. and White, S. (2001) Knowledge, truth and reflexivity: the problem of judgement in social work. *Journal of Social Work*, 1, 1.

Thagard, P. (1999) *How Scientists Explain Disease*. Princeton, NJ: Princeton University Press.

Trinder, L. (2000) Evidence-based practice in social work and probation. In L. Trinder and S. Reynolds (eds) *Evidence-based Practice: A Critical Appraisal*. Oxford: Blackwell Science.

Truman, C., Mertens, D. and Humphries, B. (eds) (2000) *Research and Inequality*. London: UCL Press.

Turk, D. C., Salovey, P. and Prentice, D. A. (1988) Psychotherapy: an information processing perspective. In D. C. Turk and P. Salovey (eds) *Reasoning, Inference and Judgement in Clinical Psychology*. New York: Free Press.

Tyson, K. (1995) *New Foundations for Scientific Social and Behavioural Research.* Boston: Allyn and Bacon.

van Zuuren, F. J. (1997) The standard of neutrality during genetic counselling: an empirical investigation. *Patient Education and Counselling*, 32, 69–79.

von Bertalannfy, L. (1971) *General Systems Theory: Foundations, Developments, Application.* London: Allen Lane.

Watzlawick, P., Beavin, J. H. and Jackson, D. D. (1967) *Pragmatics of Human Communication: A Study of Interactional Patterns, Pathologies and Paradoxes.* New York: W. W. Norton & Co.

Webb, S. (2001) Some considerations on the validity of evidence-based practice in social work. *British Journal of Social Work*, 31, 57–79.

West, C. (1996) Ethnography and orthography: a modest methodological proposal. *Journal of Contemporary Ethnography*, 25(3), 327–52.

White, S. (1997a) Beyond reproduction? Hermeneutics, reflexivity and social work practice. *British Journal of Social Work*, 27(6), 739–53.

White, S. (1997b) Performing social work: an ethnographic study of talk and text in a metropolitan social services department. Unpublished PhD thesis, University of Salford.

White, S. (1998) Interdiscursivity and child welfare: the ascent and durability of psycholegalism. *Sociological Review*, 46(2), 264–92.

White, S. (1999) Examining the artfulness of risk talk. In A. Jokinen, K. Juhila and T. Poso (eds) *Constructing Social Work Practices.* Aldershot: Ashgate.

White, S. (2001) Auto-ethnography as reflexive inquiry: the research act as self-surveillance. In I. Shaw and N. Gould (eds) *Qualitative Social Work Research: Method and Content.* London: Sage.

White, S. (2002) Accomplishing the case in paediatrics and child health: medicine and morality in interprofessional talk. *Sociology of Health and Illness*, 24(4), 409–35.

Wicks, D. (1998) *Nurses and Doctors at Work: Rethinking Professional Boundaries.* Buckingham: Open University Press.

Whyte, W. F. (1981) *Street Corner Society*, 3rd edn. Chicago: University of Chicago Press.

Wolf, F. M., Gruppen, L. D. and Billi, J. E. (1985) Differential diagnosis and competing hypotheses heuristic: a practical approach to judgement under uncertainty and Bayesian probability. *Journal of American Medical Association*, 253, 2858–62.

Wolff, G. and Young, C. (1995) Nondirectiveness and genetic counselling. *Journal of Genetic Counselling*, 4(1), 3–25.

Woodward, L., Taylor, E. and Downdney, L. (1998) The parenting and family functioning of children with hyperactivity. *Journal of Child Psychology and Psychiatry*, 39, 161–9.

Woolgar, S. (1988) Reflexivity is the ethnographer of the text. In S. Woolgar (ed.) *New Frontiers in the Sociology of Knowledge.* London: Sage.

Index

abdominal pain (Leeds study), 10
accident and emergency departments, 93–5, 97, 100
accountability, 20, 60, 130, 136–7, 146
  -neutral version (family troubles), 139, 141, 142
accounts and accounting practices, 52, 164
actor network theory, 45
acute medicine, 95–7
affective judgements, 102, 127, 128
Ahmed, W.I., 26
Alder Hey Children's Hospital, 25
Anderson, H., 131
Anspach, R., 57, 77, 97
anthropology, 49, 146, 147, 151, 153
apodictic knowledge, 66, 79, 81, 89
art-science debate, 3–23, 24, 41–2
artfulness of science, 16–22
Asperger's Syndrome, 7–8
Atkinson, P., 11, 15, 22, 45, 49, 50, 66, 68–71, 76–7, 78
attachment theory, 83–4, 148
atypical chest pain (Bayesian calculation), 11
audit (in NHS), 26, 27
Aull Davies, C., 50
authenticity, 50
authorization procedures, 50, 53, 127, 164
autism, 65
autonomy, 92, 95

backstage (in family therapy), 138–42
backward inference, 3
backward reasoning, 8
bad patients/good patients, 92, 93–5, 97–8, 99–101
Baker, T., 81
Bateson, G., 86
Bayes, Thomas, 9
Bayes' theorem, 9–13, 15, 164
'benign introspection', 19, 60, 157
Benner, P., 18
Berg, M., 4, 8, 9–10, 13
Beyth-Marom, R., 13
Billig, M., 58

biomedicine, 4, 8, 11, 15, 31, 45, 114
  formal knowledge in, 63–79
birth asphyxia, 74–5
blame
  moral judgements and, 109–12, 132–3, 136, 140
  in multidisciplinary work, 109–12
  negotiating (in interaction), 102–8
blameworthiness, 20, 91–113
blamings, 57, 99, 133, 136, 139, 156, 164
Bloor, M., 48, 50, 151, 154
body, reading/interpreting, 69–77
Boscolo, L., 130
Bosk, C.L., 78
Bowen, Jaymee, 26
Bowlby, J., 147
Bradbury, M., 48
'brain-in-a-vat' metaphor, 34–5, 149
breast beating (moral identity), 87–8
Brewer, J., 50
Bristol Royal Infirmary, 25, 35
British Journal of Social Work, 146
Brooks, L.R., 7
Brown, P., 58, 107
Brunswick, E., 12
Bryant, C.G.A., 155
bureaucratization, 25, 27
Burman, E., 60, 80
Butler-Sloss, E., 151
Buttny, R., 132

Canadian Task Force, 28
care, colonization of, 30–3
case conferences (in paediatrics), 121–8
case formulation, 40–1, 154
  approaches, 3–23
  diagnostic uncertainty, 69–77
  evidence-based practice and, 29–30, 37
  extreme, 87, 99, 166
  formal knowledge in, 63–90
  in paediatrics, 71–6, 114–29
  storytelling/persuasion in, 20–2

case study
   case formulation in paediatrics,
      114–29
   ethnographic, 49–51
categorization, 63
category bound activities (CBAs), 55–6,
      99, 100, 125
   see also membership categorization
causal explanations, 4, 5
causation, 29, 46, 114
Centre for Evidence-Based Social Services
      (University of Exeter), 146
cerebral palsy, 74–5
certainty, 8, 63, 68, 78–9, 148–9, 160
   scientific-bureaucratic model, 24–39
change of subject strategy, 133–4
Charlton, B., 41
child abuse, 36–7, 48–9, 110, 147, 151–3
child and adolescent mental health
      (CAMHS), 116
child psychiatry, 98, 110–11
children, 59
   failure to thrive, 115, 116, 117–18
   health of (moral judgement), 98–102
   -mother relationship, 6–7, 56, 99
   neonatal prognostic decision-making,
      77, 97
   'not just medical' cases, 116–28
   -parent relationships, 56, 81–8, 99–101
   at risk, 25, 35, 71–3
   voice of (privileging), 102–8, 152
   weight loss/gain, 115, 116, 117–19,
      120–2, 123–5
   see also family therapy; paediatrics
Children Act (1989), 121, 123
Cicourel, A., 14
Clarke, A., 10, 11, 144
Clavarino, A., 54, 149
Clayman, S., 130–1
Cleveland scandal, 151, 152, 153
Climbie, Victoria, 25, 35
clinical genetics, 10
clinical governance, 27, 32
clinical judgement
   approaches to understanding, 3–23
   art-science debate, 16–22
   blameworthiness and creditworthiness,
      91–113
   complexity, 37–9
   in context, 145–62
   education and training, 159–62

performing (in family therapy),
      136–8
   see also case formulation
clinical science
   popular knowledge and, 78–9
   as social practice, 63–90
clinicians
   competence (tackling error), 8–14
   use of formal knowledge, 63–90
Cochrane, A.L., 28
Cochrane Centre (Oxford), 28
Code, L., 15
cognitive-behavioural therapy, 31, 37
cognitive competence, 8–14
cognitive psychology, 3, 9
cognitive revolution, 13
cohort studies, 44
Commission for Health Improvement
      (CHI), 27
competence (tackling error), 8–14
complementarity/complementary
      interaction, 86, 88
Confidential Inquiry into Perioperative
      Death (CPoD), 108–9
confirmation bias, 13
Conservative government (1980s), 26
contrast structures, 53–4, 164
contrastive rhetoric, 109
conventional moral judgements, 94–5
conversation analysis, 57–8, 152, 164
   transcription symbols, 54, 163
   uses, 54–5
Cook, T.D., 47
Cooksy, R.W., 12
creditworthiness, 20, 91–113
crime, fear of, 43
crossover designs, 44
Cuff, E., 55, 132

Dahlberg, G., 34
Daly, J., 69
Damasio, A.R., 38, 91–2, 93, 49
Davidoff, F., 8
death
   impact of terminal illness, 59
   perioperative, 108–9
   prognostic decision-making, 77, 97
   social constructionist approach, 47–8
decision-making, 18, 37–8, 68, 77, 154, 158
   emotion and, 91, 92, 97
   hypothetico-deductive method, 6, 8, 9

inferiority of unaided, 13
support models, 15
decision analysis, 9–13, 164
de Dombal, F.T., 10
deduction/deductive reasoning, 147, 150, 165
see also hypothetico-deductive method
deep familiarity, 50, 51
deficit models, 13–14
definitional privilege, 53, 54, 165
degrees of confidence, 4
degrees of freedom, 3
Delamont, S., 66
Department of Health, 26, 27–8, 33
depressive perspective, 43
Descartes, R., 33, 38
Descartes' Error (Damasio), 91–2
developmental psychology, 116
diagnosis, 3, 63
  acute/geriatric cases, 95–7
  differential, 5
  pattern recognition, 7–8, 13, 69
  practical-moral reasoning, 78–9, 80
  uncertainty, 69–77
dialogical approach, 155–6, 162
Dingwall, R., 60, 94, 97–8, 99–100, 110, 131
discourse, 58–60, 165
discourse analysis, 3, 103, 132, 165
  Foucauldian, 58, 166
  realism in, 146, 151, 153, 156–7, 159, 162
  tacit dimension, 45, 58, 59–60
discourse studies, 58–60
discursive psychology, 58, 165
disease classification (nosologies), 4, 114, 127, 168
doctor-patient relationship, 56, 99
double-blind trials, 28, 44
Dowie, J., 13, 18, 22
Downie, R.S., 20, 29, 40–2, 150, 159–60
dramaturgical techniques, 152–3
drug metaphor, 31–3

economics, 8, 10
Eddy, D.M., 8
education, training and, 159–62
Edwards, D., 21, 47, 58
Einhorn, H.J., 3
Elstein, A.S., 7, 8, 13, 18, 22
Elwyn, G., 144, 145, 158
'embodied mind', 38, 149
emotion, 41
  morality and, 91–113

rationality and, 34, 37, 38
reason and, 34, 37, 42, 91–2, 148, 161
emotionless reason, 148
Enlightenment, 33–4, 35, 37, 165
ENT clinics, 151
epidemiology, 10–11
epistemology, 35, 165
Epstein, E., 130
equivalence paradox, 32
Eraut, M., 157
error, 8–14
esoteric knowledge, 64, 69
ethics, 41, 161–2
ethnography, 3, 16, 45, 52, 65, 98, 165–6
  case study, 49–51
  ethnomethodological, 51, 102, 166
  interactionist, 51, 167
  realism and, 146, 151, 156–7, 159, 162
ethnomethodological ethnography, 51, 102, 166
ethnomethodology, 51–5, 58, 145, 166
Eva, K.W., 7
everyday life, sociology of, 44–9, 153
evidence-based practice (EBP), 8, 25, 44, 68, 145–7, 149, 150, 161, 162
  case formulation and, 29–30, 37
  development of, 26–8
  problems/limitations, 28–33, 154–5
  protection from fads/fashions, 151–3
exoteric knowledge, 64, 66–9, 77–81, 85, 89–90, 161
experimental studies, 153–4
  observation process, 68–9
expertise, 15, 18, 29, 55
  diagnostic uncertainty, 69–77
experts, 25, 81
external evidence, 29
extreme case formulations, 87, 99, 166

factitious illness, 59
facts, 16, 24
Fahlberg, V., 83
failure to thrive, 115, 116, 117–18
falsification, 5, 46
family
  moral judgements about, 99–102
  work (moral context), 131–3
  see also children; parents
family systems therapy, 86, 88, 166

family therapy, 59–60, 58–9, 102–7, 158, 161
   neutrality in, 130–1, 132–6, 138, 143
   rhetoric and moral judgements, 130–44
feedback, 156
   in family therapy, 137, 138, 141
feminism/feminist research, 46, 154
first paradox (in family therapy), 133–6
Fischoff, B., 13
Fitzgerald, R., 55
Fleck, L., 64–6, 68–9, 73, 77, 78, 81, 149
Flynn, R., 26
formal knowledge, 63–90, 154, 160
formulation
   role/functions, 135–6, 140, 141
   see also case formulation
forward reasoning, 8
Foucauldian discourse analysis, 58, 166
Foucault, M., 58, 59, 161–2
freedom (Enlightenment thinking), 33
frontstage (in family therapy), 138–42
Frosh, S., 42, 130

Garfinkel, H., 51, 145
Garralda, M.E., 115
Geertz, C., 45
General Social Care Council, 27
genetic hypothesis, 75–6
geriatrics, 95–7, 98
germ theory of disease, 38
Giddens, A., 155–6
Glaser, B., 48
Goffman, E., 49, 92, 99, 107
Golann, S., 130
Goldberg, L.R., 12
Goldner, V., 130
Gomm, R., 28
good patients/bad patients, 92, 93–5, 97–8,
   99–101
Goolishian, H.A., 131
Graham, I., 19
grandparents (in family therapy), 86–8
Greatbatch, D., 131
Green, J., 63, 89
Greenhalgh, T., 145, 159–60
Groen, G.J., 7, 8
Grosskurth, P., 43
Gubrium, J.F., 102–3, 155
Gwyn, R., 145, 158

Hacking, I., 36, 46, 64
haematology, 69–71

Hall, C., 45, 93, 123, 129, 155
Hall, S., 148
Ham, C., 26
Hammersley, M., 45, 49, 50
handbook knowledge, 64–7, 68, 74–6,
   78–9, 85, 91, 168
Hargreaves, A., 109
Harrison, S., 24–5, 26, 29
health visitors, 110
Helicobacter pylori, 38, 66–7
heparin, 76–7
Herbert, M., 82
Higgs, Dr Marietta, 151
Hollway, W., 42–3, 51
hospitals
   accident and emergency departments,
      93–5, 97, 100
   acute medicine, 95–7
   ENT clinics, 151
   geriatric medicine, 95–7, 98
   scandals, 25, 35, 151
Housley, W., 55, 56
humanities/humaneness, 40, 41–2
Hunter, K.M., 16
Hurwitz, B., 159–60
hydronephrosis, 74
hypothesis generation/formulation,
   13–14
hypothetic-deductive method, 5–8, 9,
   45, 150, 166

impression management, 99
indifferent kinds, 36, 37, 46–7, 166
induction/inductive reasoning, 13, 16, 45,
   46, 147, 150, 166
information processing models, 9, 15
interaction (negotiating blame), 102–8
interactionist ethnography, 51, 167
interactive kinds, 36–7, 46–7, 167
interest or stake, 137, 167
interpreting the body, 69–77
interpretive social science, 146, 153,
   158
   methodologies (use of), 40–60
   paradigm, 46–7
   sociology of everyday life, 44–9
interview data/studies, 52–3, 154
'intimate knowledge', 50
intuition, 15, 16, 38–9
   tacit knowledge and, 8, 17–20, 24
intuitive reasoning, 18

Ivey, D.C., 15
Ixer, G., 20

Jayussi, L., 55
Jefferson, T., 43, 51
Jeffrey, R., 93–4, 97
John, I.D., 80, 84, 85
journal science, 64–7, 68, 69–77, 80
judgement analysis, 12–13, 167
'judgement bootstrapping', 12
'just knowing', 18

Kahneman, D., 13
Kaye, J., 32
Kennedy, J.F., 48
Kessler, S., 144
Kiesler, D.J., 31
Klein, M., 43
Knorr-Cetina, K., 35–6
know-how, 18, 39
knower-known relationship, 14–15
knowing, 33, 35
knowing-in-action, 18, 50
knowledge, 24, 44, 50, 58
    apodictic, 66, 79, 81, 89
    claims, 154, 158
    epistemology, 35, 165
    esoteric, 64, 69
    evidence-based, 25, 29, 30, 33, 34
    exoteric (popular), 64, 66–9, 77–81, 85,
        89–91, 161
    formal, 63–90, 154, 160
    -in-action, 18, 150
    making, 136–8, 154, 159
    realism and, 14–15
    tacit, 8, 17–20, 24, 52, 157, 168
    theoretical, 80–90
    to go (vade mecum), 64–7, 68, 74–6, 78–9,
        85, 91, 168
Kuhn, T., 64

laboratory science (producing and
    distributing), 64–8
language, 6, 8, 15, 20, 52
    see also conversation analysis
Lannamann, J.W., 132
Latimer, J., 45, 95–7, 98
Latour, B., 34–5, 37, 38, 149–50, 155, 161
Launer, J., 159, 161
Levinson, S.C., 58, 108
literature, truth in, 41–2

Little, M., 4, 6, 11, 12, 20, 40, 41–2, 145
Lloyd, R.M., 103, 151, 152–3
Loos, V.E., 130
Lucey, C., 81

Macdonald, G., 146
MacDonald, G.M., 31
McHugh, P., 94
Macnaughton, J., 20, 29, 40, 41, 42, 150,
    159–60
McNeish, D., 145
Malinowski, B., 45
Marks, D., 58, 60
Marxism, 153, 154
Mary Eminson scale, 125
mathematics, 3, 8
May, C., 34, 59
Maynard, D., 51–2
Meadow, R., 59
meaning-making, 20, 22
measles, mumps and rubella vaccine,
    146
medical model, 161
medicine, 4, 8
membership categorization, 55–8, 99, 108,
    167
membership categorization devices (MCDs),
    56, 167
men, see family; family therapy; parents
mental illness, 36, 52–3
meta-analyses, 28
metaphors, 13, 31–5, 42, 149
methodologies
    interpretive social science, 40–60, 146,
        153
    qualitative research, 45, 153–4
minimal response tokens, 136, 167
Mishler, E.G., 21
Mitchell, J.C., 50
Mitchie, S., 144
MMR vaccine, 146
modernity, 33–4, 161, 167
moral context (family work), 131–3
moral identity, 87–8
moral judgements, 37, 38
    blame and, 110–12
    child health and, 98–102
    emotion and, 91, 92–6, 100–2
    formal knowledge and, 78–81
    organizational context and, 95–9
    in paediatrics, 114–29

practical-moral reasoning, 78–9, 80, 93, 136, 137, 138
  rhetoric and, 130–44
moral self/selves, 108–12
morality
  emotion and, 91–113
  moral dimension of talk, 55–8
  in paediatrics, 114–29
mother-child relationship, 6–7, 56, 99
Mulkay, M., 35–6
multidimensionality, 31
multidisciplinary work, 110–12
multiple versions (in family therapy case), 130–44
Munchausen syndrome by proxy, 59, 117, 122–3, 124, 127
Murphy, E., 153, 154
Murray, T., 60, 94, 97–8, 99–100

narratives, 20–1, 43, 167
National Care Standards Commission, 27–8
National Health Service, 25, 27
  multidisciplinary work, 110–12
  Research and Development initiative, 26, 28
  see also hospitals
National Institute for Clinical Excellence (NICE), 27
natural sciences, 34, 35
neonatal paediatrics, 75–6, 77, 97
neutrality, 156
  in family therapy, 130–1, 132, 133–6, 138, 142
New, B., 26
New Labour government, 26–7
news interviewing (neutrality), 130–1
NHS Executive, 27
non-accidental injury, 71
non-conventional moral judgement, 94–5
non-lexical vocalizations, 54
'normal science', 64
Norman, G.R., 8
normative judgements, 46
nosologies, 4, 114, 127, 168
'not just medical' cases, 116–28
'not knowing' position, 130, 131, 132
nursing study, 95–8

objective reasoning, 16, 19, 24
objectivity, 33, 34, 37

observation
  of human relationships, 80–90
  process, 68–9
  psychological theory and, 80–90
oppression, 46, 154
organizational context, moral judgements and, 95–9
orthopaedics, 72–3
outcomes, 29–30, 32
Owen, I.R., 31, 32

paediatrics, 16, 65, 98
  diagnostic uncertainty, 71–6
  membership categorization, 56–7
  multidisciplinary work, 110–11
  neonatal, 75–6, 77, 97
  'not just medica' cases, 116–28
  outpatients clinic, 108–9
  practical-moral reasoning, 78–9
  science, morality and case formulation in, 114–29
  see also children
paradigms/paradigm-specific concepts, 64
paranoid-schizoid perspective, 43
parenting, 81, 100, 116, 125
parents
  attributing blame to, 102–8
  -child relationship, 56, 81–8, 99–101
  love, child health and, 98–102
  in 'not just medical' cases, 116–28
  -professionals interaction, 95
Parry, G., 33
Parsloe, P., 80
Pasveer, B., 69
Patel, V.L., 7, 8
pathology, 69–71
patients
  doctors and (relationship), 56, 99
  good/bad, 92, 93–5, 97–8, 99–101
  nursing responses, 95–8
pattern recognition, 7–8, 13, 69
perioperative death, 108–9
persuasion, 15, 20–2, 141
Peters, R.S., 159
philosophy, 63
Piaget, J., 147
Polanyi, M., 17
policy
  current initiatives, 24–39
  research and (connections), 155–6
political pragmatism, 26–8

Pollitt, C., 26
Pomerantz, A.M., 99, 111
Popper, Karl, 5–8
popular knowledge, 64, 66–9, 77–81, 85, 90, 161
positive connotation, 86
positivist paradigm, 46–7
post-traumatic stress disorder, 84–5
Potter, J., 21, 47, 58, 80, 135
practical-moral reasoning, 78–9, 80, 93, 136, 137, 138
practice, research and (connecting), 155–6
preferences, subjective, 11
prescriptive judgements, 46
probability theory, 8, 9–13, 14, 29
problem-solving, 17
process, outcomes and, 32
professional narratives, 20–1, 167
professional scandals, 25, 35, 151
professionals, formal knowledge used by, 63–90
prognosis/prognosis statements, 58, 59
progress, modernity and, 33–4, 161
protamine, 76
psychiatry
  child, 98, 110–11
  clinical practice, 78–9
psychoanalysis, 42–4, 45
psychodynamic theory, 89
psychological theory, 80–90
psychology, 3, 9
  discursive, 58, 165
psychopharmacological research, 31–3
psychosocial cases, 37, 59, 98–9, 114–16, 118–19
psychosomatic symptoms, 96
psychotherapy, 5, 31–3, 34, 37, 44
purchaser-provider split, 26

qualitative research, 45, 153–4
quasi-market principles, 26

radiology, 71–3
randomized controlled trial (RCT), 28, 29, 30, 33, 44, 146, 150, 154
rational-technical approach, 14, 17, 26
rationality, 42
  scientific-bureaucratic model, 24–39
  see also reason; reasoning
rationing (of health care), 26, 33

reading
  the body, 69–77
  relationships, 80–90
realism, 14–15, 168
  clinical judgement in context, 145–62
  Enlightenment version, 33, 35
  science and, 148–50
reality, 33, 36, 38, 45, 58
reason
  emotion and, 34, 37, 42, 91–2, 148, 161
  Enlightenment movement, 33–4, 37
  modernity and, 33–4, 161
  see also rationality; reasoning
reasoning, 3, 5, 8–9, 12
  deductive, 147, 150, 165
  embodied mind, 38, 149
  inductive, 13, 16, 45, 46, 147, 150, 166
  intuitive, 18
  objective, 16, 19, 24
  practical-moral, 78–9, 80, 93, 136, 137, 138
recapitulation (narrative), 21
Reder, P., 81
reflection (definitions), 157
reflection-in-action, 17–18
reflection-on-action, 17, 18, 19, 42, 51, 156–9
reflective practice/practitioner, 19–20, 42, 157
reflex anal dilatation, 151
reflexivity, 156–9, 160, 161
reframing (positive connotation), 86
Reichardt, C.S., 47
Reissman, C.K., 21, 43
relationships
  mother-child, 6–7, 56, 99
  parent-child, 56, 81–8, 99–101
  reading, 80–90
relativism, 35–6, 149, 151, 168
research
  practice and (connecting), 155–6
  qualitative, 45, 153–4
  tacit dimension, 40–60
Research and Development initiative (of NHS), 26, 28
resource allocation, 30
  rationing, 26, 33
rhetoric, 21, 168
  moral judgement and, 130–44
rhetoric of deliberate vagueness, 140, 168
Richardson, A., 33
Rolfe, G., 18, 20

Rose, N., 60
rule-breaking behaviour, 93–4

Sackett, D.L., 29, 145
Sacks, H., 54, 55, 145
Salter-Ainsworth, M., 147
scandals (in UK), 25, 35, 151
Schön, D.A., 17–18, 39, 42, 50, 156
Schwartz, A., 7, 13
science, 37–8, 146–7
  -art debate, 3–23
  artfulness of, 16–22
  case formulation and (paediatrics),
    114–29
  journal, 64–7, 68, 69–77, 80
  modernity and, 33–4
  producing and distributing, 64–8
  realism and, 148–50
  see also natural sciences; social science
'science wars', 148–50
scientific-bureaucratic model, 24–39, 44
scientific method, 4–8
scientists, professional socialization of, 66
second paradox (in family therapy), 136–8
self, moral, 107–12
Self, W., 80
self-knowledge, 42–4
self-reflexivity, 158
semiotics, 45
Shapiro, D.A., 31, 32
Sheldon, B., 31, 146–51, 153
Sheppard, M., 5, 6–7
Shipman, Harold, 25, 35
Shotter, J., 58
'significant harm', 121, 122, 127
Silverman, D., 45, 46, 48, 51, 54, 55, 95, 115,
    117, 153–4, 155
single case experiment, 44
Slembrook, S., 123, 129
Smith, D., 52–4, 125
social care, 5, 6, 15, 85–9, 145–6
  multidisciplinary work, 110–12
  scientific-bureaucratic model, 27–8, 30–1
Social Care Institute for Excellence (SCIE), 27,
    28
social constructionism, 35, 36, 38, 47–8, 168
social context, 20, 21, 41
social engineering model, 155
social judgement theory, 12–13, 167
social learning theory, 82–3, 84
social reality, 58

social science
  interpretive, *see* interpretive social science
  research/practice, 155–6
social services (multidisciplinary work),
    111–12
social worker
  in family therapy session, 103–7
  therapy session discussion, 85–9
sociological inquiry (uses/abuses), 153–5
sociology, 147
  of everyday life, 44–9, 153
somatic symptoms, 96
special study modules, 160
Stainton Rogers, R., 60
Stainton Rogers, W., 60
stake or interest, 137, 167
Stancombe, J., 15, 31, 32, 59, 95, 103, 133
standardization, 34
standardized relational pairs (SRPs), 56, 99,
    168
Stanley, L., 46
'state-counsellor' model, 155
statistics/statistical models, 8, 9, 10–13, 14,
    24, 33, 37
Stevenson, O., 80
Stiles, W.B., 31, 32
storytelling, 15, 43, 100, 109, 115–16
  in case formulation, 20–2
  in clinical practice, 58–60
Strauss, A., 48
Strong, P., 45, 100, 118–19, 128, 145
subconscious, 42–3
subjective preferences, 11
subjective probabilities, 11, 12
subjectivity, 16, 19, 24
Sudnow, D., 48

tacit dimension (research), 40–60
tacit knowledge, 8, 17–20, 24, 52, 157, 168
talk, 52, 53–4
  moral dimension, 55–8
  neutrality in, 130–1, 133–6
  see also conversation analysis
'talking cure, 31
Taylor, C., 15, 18–20, 35, 52, 95, 110, 148,
    154, 156–7, 159, 161
technical rationality, 14, 17, 26
technology of biomedicine, 69–77
television news interviewing
  (neutrality in), 130–1
terminal illness, 59

Thagard, P., 38, 66–7
theoretical knowledge, 80–90
theoreticity concept, 94
theory-driven observations, 147–8
therapeutics, 15, 30–1, 85–9
'thick description', 45, 49
third paradox (in family therapy),
    138–42
thought style, 64
training, education and, 159–62
Trainspotting (film), 42
transcription symbols, 54, 163
treatments, outcomes and, 29–30
Trinder, L., 31
Truman, C., 46
truth, 33, 34, 38, 41–2, 85
    realism and, 14–15
    regimes of, 58

uncertainty, 8, 16, 17, 24, 68, 91
    formal knowledge and, 69–81, 160
    practical-moral reasoning, 78–9, 80
    reading the body, 69–77
unconscious, 42–3
utility theory, 10, 11, 12, 45, 155

vade mecum, 64–7, 68, 74–6, 85, 90, 168
value judgements, 10

van Zuuren, F.J., 144
victimization (in families), 136–8, 140

Watzlawick, P., 86
'ways to stray', 13–14
Webb, S., 44–5, 146, 148
weight loss/gain (child development), 115,
    116, 117–19, 120–2, 123–5
West, C., 54
Wetherell, M., 21
White, S., 7, 15, 18–20, 31–2, 35, 45, 50, 52,
    56–7, 60, 80–1, 95, 98, 103, 107, 110,
    115–16, 148, 151–2, 154, 156–7, 159,
    161
Whyte, W.F., 45
Williams, G., 26
Wolf, F.M., 13
Wolff, G., 144
women
    feminism/feminist research, 46, 154
    mother-child relationship, 6–7, 56, 99
    see also family; family therapy; parents
Woodward, L., 115
Woolgar, S., 19, 157

Young, C., 144

zone of relevance, 57, 128

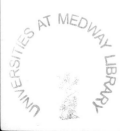